MY DIET AND EXERCISE JOURNAL

Pamela McCallum
CONVERPAGE Digital Reproductions

Before starting any diet or exercise program it is
recommended that you consult your physician.

ISBN: 0-9820733-2-1

Digitally reproduced in 2008 by:
CONVERPAGE
23 Acorn Street
Scituate, MA 02066
www.converpage.com

REASONS WHY YOU SHOULD RECORD
EVERYTHING YOU EAT:

By monitoring how many calories, fat or carbohydrates you take in each day you can begin to decrease these amounts and lose weight.

By recording what you eat it helps you decide what food groups you are missing. Many people don't eat the recommended fruits and vegetables to meet a healthy diet. Writing down the foods you eat helps you see what you are missing and meet those requirements.

Creating a record of your daily food intake and exercise program can be very beneficial to your physician if he prescribes a special diet for you.

Knowing you have to write down what you eat may make you stop the urge to eat unhealthy foods.

You can see great progress by looking back at your records at what you have accomplished in your strive to eat healthy.

Many people can suffer with medical problems based on their diet. By recording what you eat helps you discover problem foods and what you should avoid.

Recording your food intake makes you realize just how much food you are eating each day.

TABLE OF CONTENTS

DAY 1

FOOD TRACKING

DESCRIPTION

**CALORIE/
FAT/CARB**

_____   _____

_____   _____

_____   _____

_____   _____

_____   _____

_____   _____

_____   _____

_____   _____

_____   _____

_____   _____

_____   _____

_____   _____

_____   _____

_____   _____

_____   _____

TOTALS   _____

GLASSES OF WATER CHECK-LIST

☐   ☐   ☐   ☐

☐   ☐   ☐   ☐

DAILY EXERCISES (SEE EXERCISE LIST)

DESCRIPTION   **TIME**

_____   _____

_____   _____

_____   _____

_____   _____

_____   _____

_____   _____

NOTES

_____

_____

_____

_____

_____

_____

_____

DAY 2

FOOD TRACKING

DESCRIPTION	CALORIE/ FAT/CARB
_____	_____
_____	_____
_____	_____
_____	_____
_____	_____
_____	_____
_____	_____
_____	_____
_____	_____
_____	_____
_____	_____
_____	_____
_____	_____
_____	_____
_____	_____
_____	_____

TOTALS _____

GLASSES OF WATER CHECK-LIST

☐ ☐ ☐ ☐

☐ ☐ ☐ ☐

DAILY EXERCISES (SEE EXERCISE LIST)

DESCRIPTION	TIME
_____	____
_____	____
_____	____
_____	____
_____	____

NOTES

_____

_____

_____

_____

_____

_____

_____

DAY 3

FOOD TRACKING

DESCRIPTION   **CALORIE/**
                           FAT/CARB

_____   _____

_____   _____

_____   _____

_____   _____

_____   _____

_____   _____

_____   _____

_____   _____

_____   _____

_____   _____

_____   _____

_____   _____

_____   _____

_____   _____

_____   _____

_____   _____

TOTALS   _____

GLASSES OF WATER CHECK-LIST

☐   ☐   ☐   ☐

☐   ☐   ☐   ☐

DAILY EXERCISES (SEE EXERCISE LIST)

DESCRIPTION   **TIME**

_____   _____

_____   _____

_____   _____

_____   _____

_____   _____

_____   _____

NOTES

_____

_____

_____

_____

_____

_____

_____

DAY 4

FOOD TRACKING

GLASSES OF WATER CHECK-LIST

DESCRIPTION	CALORIE/ FAT/CARB
_____	_____
_____	_____
_____	_____
_____	_____
_____	_____
_____	_____
_____	_____
_____	_____
_____	_____
_____	_____
_____	_____
_____	_____
_____	_____
_____	_____
_____	_____
_____	_____
_____	_____

☐ ☐ ☐ ☐
☐ ☐ ☐ ☐

DAILY EXERCISES (SEE EXERCISE LIST)

DESCRIPTION	TIME
_____	_____
_____	_____
_____	_____
_____	_____
_____	_____
_____	_____

NOTES

_____
_____
_____
_____
_____
_____
_____

TOTALS _____

DAY 5

FOOD TRACKING

DESCRIPTION	CALORIE/ FAT/CARB
_____	_____
_____	_____
_____	_____
_____	_____
_____	_____
_____	_____
_____	_____
_____	_____
_____	_____
_____	_____
_____	_____
_____	_____
_____	_____
_____	_____
_____	_____
_____	_____

TOTALS _____

GLASSES OF WATER CHECK-LIST

☐ ☐ ☐ ☐

☐ ☐ ☐ ☐

DAILY EXERCISES (SEE EXERCISE LIST)

DESCRIPTION	TIME
_____	____
_____	____
_____	____
_____	____
_____	____
_____	____

NOTES

_____
_____
_____
_____
_____
_____
_____

DAY 6

FOOD TRACKING

DESCRIPTION	CALORIE/ FAT/CARB
_____	_____
_____	_____
_____	_____
_____	_____
_____	_____
_____	_____
_____	_____
_____	_____
_____	_____
_____	_____
_____	_____
_____	_____
_____	_____
_____	_____
_____	_____
_____	_____
_____	_____

TOTALS _____

GLASSES OF WATER CHECK-LIST

☐ ☐ ☐ ☐

☐ ☐ ☐ ☐

DAILY EXERCISES (SEE EXERCISE LIST)

DESCRIPTION	TIME
_____	_____
_____	_____
_____	_____
_____	_____
_____	_____
_____	_____

NOTES

_____

_____

_____

_____

_____

_____

_____

DAY 7

FOOD TRACKING

DESCRIPTION	CALORIE/ FAT/CARB
_____	_____
_____	_____
_____	_____
_____	_____
_____	_____
_____	_____
_____	_____
_____	_____
_____	_____
_____	_____
_____	_____
_____	_____
_____	_____
_____	_____
_____	_____
_____	_____
_____	_____

TOTALS _____

GLASSES OF WATER CHECK-LIST

☐ ☐ ☐ ☐

☐ ☐ ☐ ☐

DAILY EXERCISES (SEE EXERCISE LIST)

DESCRIPTION	TIME
_____	_____
_____	_____
_____	_____
_____	_____
_____	_____
_____	_____

NOTES

_____

_____

_____

_____

_____

_____

_____

WEEKLY TOTALS

	CALORIES FAT OR CARBS	WATER	EXERCISE TIME
DAY 1	_____	_____	_____
DAY 2	_____	_____	_____
DAY 3	_____	_____	_____
DAY 4	_____	_____	_____
DAY 5	_____	_____	_____
DAY 6	_____	_____	_____
DAY 7	_____	_____	_____
TOTALS	_____	_____	_____

DAY 1

FOOD TRACKING

DESCRIPTION	CALORIE/ FAT/CARB
_____	_____
_____	_____
_____	_____
_____	_____
_____	_____
_____	_____
_____	_____
_____	_____
_____	_____
_____	_____
_____	_____
_____	_____
_____	_____
_____	_____
_____	_____
_____	_____

GLASSES OF WATER CHECK-LIST

☐   ☐   ☐   ☐

☐   ☐   ☐   ☐

DAILY EXERCISES (SEE EXERCISE LIST)

DESCRIPTION	TIME
_____	_____
_____	_____
_____	_____
_____	_____
_____	_____
_____	_____

NOTES

_____

_____

_____

_____

_____

_____

_____

TOTALS _____

DAY 2

FOOD TRACKING

DESCRIPTION	CALORIE/ FAT/CARB
_____	_____
_____	_____
_____	_____
_____	_____
_____	_____
_____	_____
_____	_____
_____	_____
_____	_____
_____	_____
_____	_____
_____	_____
_____	_____
_____	_____
_____	_____
_____	_____

TOTALS _____

GLASSES OF WATER CHECK-LIST

☐ ☐ ☐ ☐

☐ ☐ ☐ ☐

DAILY EXERCISES (SEE EXERCISE LIST)

DESCRIPTION	TIME
_____	_____
_____	_____
_____	_____
_____	_____
_____	_____
_____	_____

NOTES

_____

_____

_____

_____

_____

_____

_____

DAY 3

FOOD TRACKING

DESCRIPTION	CALORIE/ FAT/CARB
_____	_____
_____	_____
_____	_____
_____	_____
_____	_____
_____	_____
_____	_____
_____	_____
_____	_____
_____	_____
_____	_____
_____	_____
_____	_____
_____	_____
_____	_____
_____	_____

TOTALS _____

GLASSES OF WATER CHECK-LIST

☐ ☐ ☐ ☐

☐ ☐ ☐ ☐

DAILY EXERCISES (SEE EXERCISE LIST)

DESCRIPTION	TIME
_____	_____
_____	_____
_____	_____
_____	_____
_____	_____
_____	_____

NOTES

_____

_____

_____

_____

_____

_____

_____

DAY 4

FOOD TRACKING

DESCRIPTION   **CALORIE/
                                FAT/CARB**

_____   _____

_____   _____

_____   _____

_____   _____

_____   _____

_____   _____

_____   _____

_____   _____

_____   _____

_____   _____

_____   _____

_____   _____

_____   _____

_____   _____

_____   _____

_____   _____

TOTALS   _____

GLASSES OF WATER CHECK-LIST

☐   ☐   ☐   ☐

☐   ☐   ☐   ☐

DAILY EXERCISES (SEE EXERCISE LIST)

DESCRIPTION   **TIME**

_____   _____

_____   _____

_____   _____

_____   _____

_____   _____

_____   _____

NOTES

_____

_____

_____

_____

_____

_____

_____

DAY 5

FOOD TRACKING

DESCRIPTION	CALORIE/ FAT/CARB
_____	_____
_____	_____
_____	_____
_____	_____
_____	_____
_____	_____
_____	_____
_____	_____
_____	_____
_____	_____
_____	_____
_____	_____
_____	_____
_____	_____
_____	_____
_____	_____
_____	_____
_____	_____

TOTALS _____

GLASSES OF WATER CHECK-LIST

☐ ☐ ☐ ☐

☐ ☐ ☐ ☐

DAILY EXERCISES (SEE EXERCISE LIST)

DESCRIPTION	TIME
_____	____
_____	____
_____	____
_____	____
_____	____
_____	____

NOTES

_____

_____

_____

_____

_____

_____

_____

_____

19

DAY 6

FOOD TRACKING

DESCRIPTION	CALORIE/ FAT/CARB
_____	_____
_____	_____
_____	_____
_____	_____
_____	_____
_____	_____
_____	_____
_____	_____
_____	_____
_____	_____
_____	_____
_____	_____
_____	_____
_____	_____
_____	_____
_____	_____
_____	_____

TOTALS _____

GLASSES OF WATER CHECK-LIST

☐ ☐ ☐ ☐

☐ ☐ ☐ ☐

DAILY EXERCISES (SEE EXERCISE LIST)

DESCRIPTION	TIME
_____	_____
_____	_____
_____	_____
_____	_____
_____	_____

NOTES

_____

_____

_____

_____

_____

_____

_____

DAY 7

FOOD TRACKING

DESCRIPTION	CALORIE/ FAT/CARB
_____	_____
_____	_____
_____	_____
_____	_____
_____	_____
_____	_____
_____	_____
_____	_____
_____	_____
_____	_____
_____	_____
_____	_____
_____	_____
_____	_____
_____	_____
_____	_____
_____	_____
_____	_____

TOTALS _____

GLASSES OF WATER CHECK-LIST

☐ ☐ ☐ ☐

☐ ☐ ☐ ☐

DAILY EXERCISES (SEE EXERCISE LIST)

DESCRIPTION	TIME
_____	____
_____	____
_____	____
_____	____
_____	____
_____	____

NOTES

_____

_____

_____

_____

_____

_____

_____

WEEKLY TOTALS

	CALORIES FAT OR CARBS	WATER	EXERCISE TIME
DAY 1	_____	_____	_____
DAY 2	_____	_____	_____
DAY 3	_____	_____	_____
DAY 4	_____	_____	_____
DAY 5	_____	_____	_____
DAY 6	_____	_____	_____
DAY 7	_____	_____	_____
TOTALS	_____	_____	_____

DAY 1

FOOD TRACKING

DESCRIPTION   CALORIE/
                              FAT/CARB

_____ _____

_____ _____

_____ _____

_____ _____

_____ _____

_____ _____

_____ _____

_____ _____

_____ _____

_____ _____

_____ _____

_____ _____

_____ _____

_____ _____

_____ _____

_____ _____

TOTALS   _____

GLASSES OF WATER CHECK-LIST

☐   ☐   ☐   ☐

☐   ☐   ☐   ☐

DAILY EXERCISES (SEE EXERCISE LIST)

DESCRIPTION   TIME

_____ _____

_____ _____

_____ _____

_____ _____

_____ _____

_____ _____

NOTES

_____

_____

_____

_____

_____

_____

_____

DAY 2

FOOD TRACKING

DESCRIPTION	CALORIE/ FAT/CARB
_____	_____
_____	_____
_____	_____
_____	_____
_____	_____
_____	_____
_____	_____
_____	_____
_____	_____
_____	_____
_____	_____
_____	_____
_____	_____
_____	_____
_____	_____

TOTALS _____

GLASSES OF WATER CHECK-LIST

☐ ☐ ☐ ☐

☐ ☐ ☐ ☐

DAILY EXERCISES (SEE EXERCISE LIST)

DESCRIPTION	TIME
_____	____
_____	____
_____	____
_____	____
_____	____
_____	____

NOTES

_____

_____

_____

_____

_____

_____

_____

DAY 3

FOOD TRACKING

DESCRIPTION   **CALORIE/**
                        FAT/CARB

_____   _____

_____   _____

_____   _____

_____   _____

_____   _____

_____   _____

_____   _____

_____   _____

_____   _____

_____   _____

_____   _____

_____   _____

_____   _____

_____   _____

_____   _____

_____   _____

_____   _____

TOTALS   _____

GLASSES OF WATER CHECK-LIST

☐   ☐   ☐   ☐

☐   ☐   ☐   ☐

DAILY EXERCISES (SEE EXERCISE LIST)

DESCRIPTION   **TIME**

_____   _____

_____   _____

_____   _____

_____   _____

_____   _____

_____   _____

NOTES

_____

_____

_____

_____

_____

_____

_____

DAY 4

FOOD TRACKING

DESCRIPTION	CALORIE/ FAT/CARB
_____	_____
_____	_____
_____	_____
_____	_____
_____	_____
_____	_____
_____	_____
_____	_____
_____	_____
_____	_____
_____	_____
_____	_____
_____	_____
_____	_____
_____	_____
_____	_____
_____	_____

TOTALS _____

GLASSES OF WATER CHECK-LIST

☐　　☐　　☐　　☐

☐　　☐　　☐　　☐

DAILY EXERCISES (SEE EXERCISE LIST)

DESCRIPTION	TIME
_____	_____
_____	_____
_____	_____
_____	_____
_____	_____
_____	_____

NOTES

_____

_____

_____

_____

_____

_____

_____

DAY 5

FOOD TRACKING

DESCRIPTION   **CALORIE/**
                         FAT/CARB

_____ _____

_____ _____

_____ _____

_____ _____

_____ _____

_____ _____

_____ _____

_____ _____

_____ _____

_____ _____

_____ _____

_____ _____

_____ _____

_____ _____

_____ _____

_____ _____

_____ _____

_____ _____

TOTALS   _____

GLASSES OF WATER CHECK-LIST

☐   ☐   ☐   ☐

☐   ☐   ☐   ☐

DAILY EXERCISES (SEE EXERCISE LIST)

DESCRIPTION   **TIME**

_____ _____

_____ _____

_____ _____

_____ _____

_____ _____

_____ _____

NOTES

_____

_____

_____

_____

_____

_____

_____

DAY 6

FOOD TRACKING

DESCRIPTION   **CALORIE/ FAT/CARB**

_____   _____

_____   _____

_____   _____

_____   _____

_____   _____

_____   _____

_____   _____

_____   _____

_____   _____

_____   _____

_____   _____

_____   _____

_____   _____

_____   _____

_____   _____

_____   _____

_____   _____

TOTALS   _____

GLASSES OF WATER CHECK-LIST

☐   ☐   ☐   ☐

☐   ☐   ☐   ☐

DAILY EXERCISES (SEE EXERCISE LIST)

DESCRIPTION   **TIME**

_____   _____

_____   _____

_____   _____

_____   _____

_____   _____

_____   _____

NOTES

_____

_____

_____

_____

_____

_____

_____

DAY 7

FOOD TRACKING

DESCRIPTION   **CALORIE/**
                         FAT/CARB

_____ _____

_____ _____

_____ _____

_____ _____

_____ _____

_____ _____

_____ _____

_____ _____

_____ _____

_____ _____

_____ _____

_____ _____

_____ _____

_____ _____

_____ _____

_____ _____

_____ _____

TOTALS   _____

GLASSES OF WATER CHECK-LIST

☐   ☐   ☐   ☐

☐   ☐   ☐   ☐

DAILY EXERCISES (SEE EXERCISE LIST)

DESCRIPTION   **TIME**

_____ _____

_____ _____

_____ _____

_____ _____

_____ _____

_____ _____

NOTES

_____

_____

_____

_____

_____

_____

_____

WEEKLY TOTALS

	CALORIES FAT OR CARBS	WATER	EXERCISE TIME
DAY 1	_____	_____	_____
DAY 2	_____	_____	_____
DAY 3	_____	_____	_____
DAY 4	_____	_____	_____
DAY 5	_____	_____	_____
DAY 6	_____	_____	_____
DAY 7	_____	_____	_____
TOTALS	_____	_____	_____

DAY 1

FOOD TRACKING

DESCRIPTION   CALORIE/
                          FAT/CARB

_____ _____

_____ _____

_____ _____

_____ _____

_____ _____

_____ _____

_____ _____

_____ _____

_____ _____

_____ _____

_____ _____

_____ _____

_____ _____

_____ _____

_____ _____

_____ _____

_____ _____

TOTALS   _____

GLASSES OF WATER CHECK-LIST

☐ ☐ ☐ ☐

☐ ☐ ☐ ☐

DAILY EXERCISES (SEE EXERCISE LIST)

DESCRIPTION   TIME

_____ ____

_____ ____

_____ ____

_____ ____

_____ ____

_____ ____

NOTES

_____

_____

_____

_____

_____

_____

_____

_____

DAY 2

FOOD TRACKING

DESCRIPTION	CALORIE/ FAT/CARB
_____	_____
_____	_____
_____	_____
_____	_____
_____	_____
_____	_____
_____	_____
_____	_____
_____	_____
_____	_____
_____	_____
_____	_____
_____	_____
_____	_____
_____	_____
_____	_____
_____	_____
_____	_____

TOTALS _____

GLASSES OF WATER CHECK-LIST

☐ ☐ ☐ ☐

☐ ☐ ☐ ☐

DAILY EXERCISES (SEE EXERCISE LIST)

DESCRIPTION	TIME
_____	____
_____	____
_____	____
_____	____
_____	____
_____	____

NOTES

_____

_____

_____

_____

_____

_____

_____

DAY 3

FOOD TRACKING

DESCRIPTION   CALORIE/
                               FAT/CARB

_____ _____

_____ _____

_____ _____

_____ _____

_____ _____

_____ _____

_____ _____

_____ _____

_____ _____

_____ _____

_____ _____

_____ _____

_____ _____

_____ _____

_____ _____

_____ _____

TOTALS   _____

GLASSES OF WATER CHECK-LIST

☐   ☐   ☐   ☐

☐   ☐   ☐   ☐

DAILY EXERCISES (SEE EXERCISE LIST)

DESCRIPTION   TIME

_____ ____

_____ ____

_____ ____

_____ ____

_____ ____

NOTES

_____

_____

_____

_____

_____

_____

_____

DAY 4

FOOD TRACKING

DESCRIPTION	CALORIE/ FAT/CARB
_____	_____
_____	_____
_____	_____
_____	_____
_____	_____
_____	_____
_____	_____
_____	_____
_____	_____
_____	_____
_____	_____
_____	_____
_____	_____
_____	_____
_____	_____
_____	_____
_____	_____
_____	_____

TOTALS _____

GLASSES OF WATER CHECK-LIST

☐ ☐ ☐ ☐

☐ ☐ ☐ ☐

DAILY EXERCISES (SEE EXERCISE LIST)

DESCRIPTION	TIME
_____	_____
_____	_____
_____	_____
_____	_____
_____	_____
_____	_____

NOTES

_____

_____

_____

_____

_____

_____

_____

DAY 5

FOOD TRACKING

DESCRIPTION	CALORIE/ FAT/CARB
_____	_____
_____	_____
_____	_____
_____	_____
_____	_____
_____	_____
_____	_____
_____	_____
_____	_____
_____	_____
_____	_____
_____	_____
_____	_____
_____	_____
_____	_____
_____	_____
_____	_____

TOTALS _____

GLASSES OF WATER CHECK-LIST

☐   ☐   ☐   ☐

☐   ☐   ☐   ☐

DAILY EXERCISES (SEE EXERCISE LIST)

DESCRIPTION	TIME
_____	____
_____	____
_____	____
_____	____
_____	____
_____	____

NOTES

_____

_____

_____

_____

_____

_____

_____

DAY 6

FOOD TRACKING

DESCRIPTION	CALORIE/ FAT/CARB
_____	_____
_____	_____
_____	_____
_____	_____
_____	_____
_____	_____
_____	_____
_____	_____
_____	_____
_____	_____
_____	_____
_____	_____
_____	_____
_____	_____
_____	_____
_____	_____
_____	_____

TOTALS _____

GLASSES OF WATER CHECK-LIST

☐ ☐ ☐ ☐

☐ ☐ ☐ ☐

DAILY EXERCISES (SEE EXERCISE LIST)

DESCRIPTION	TIME
_____	_____
_____	_____
_____	_____
_____	_____
_____	_____
_____	_____

NOTES

_____

_____

_____

_____

_____

_____

_____

DAY 7

FOOD TRACKING

DESCRIPTION	CALORIE/ FAT/CARB
_____	_____
_____	_____
_____	_____
_____	_____
_____	_____
_____	_____
_____	_____
_____	_____
_____	_____
_____	_____
_____	_____
_____	_____
_____	_____
_____	_____
_____	_____
_____	_____
_____	_____

TOTALS _____

GLASSES OF WATER CHECK-LIST

☐ ☐ ☐ ☐

☐ ☐ ☐ ☐

DAILY EXERCISES (SEE EXERCISE LIST)

DESCRIPTION	TIME
_____	____
_____	____
_____	____
_____	____
_____	____
_____	____

NOTES

_____

_____

_____

_____

_____

_____

_____

WEEKLY TOTALS

	CALORIES FAT OR CARBS	WATER	EXERCISE TIME
DAY 1	_____	_____	_____
DAY 2	_____	_____	_____
DAY 3	_____	_____	_____
DAY 4	_____	_____	_____
DAY 5	_____	_____	_____
DAY 6	_____	_____	_____
DAY 7	_____	_____	_____
TOTALS	_____	_____	_____

DAY 1

FOOD TRACKING

DESCRIPTION   **CALORIE/**
                         FAT/CARB

_____ _____

_____ _____

_____ _____

_____ _____

_____ _____

_____ _____

_____ _____

_____ _____

_____ _____

_____ _____

_____ _____

_____ _____

_____ _____

_____ _____

_____ _____

_____ _____

_____ _____

TOTALS   _____

GLASSES OF WATER CHECK-LIST

☐   ☐   ☐   ☐

☐   ☐   ☐   ☐

DAILY EXERCISES (SEE EXERCISE LIST)

DESCRIPTION   **TIME**

_____ _____

_____ _____

_____ _____

_____ _____

_____ _____

_____ _____

NOTES

_____

_____

_____

_____

_____

_____

_____

DAY 2

FOOD TRACKING

DESCRIPTION   **CALORIE/ FAT/CARB**

_____ _____

_____ _____

_____ _____

_____ _____

_____ _____

_____ _____

_____ _____

_____ _____

_____ _____

_____ _____

_____ _____

_____ _____

_____ _____

_____ _____

_____ _____

_____ _____

TOTALS   _____

GLASSES OF WATER CHECK-LIST

☐ ☐ ☐ ☐

☐ ☐ ☐ ☐

DAILY EXERCISES (SEE EXERCISE LIST)

DESCRIPTION   **TIME**

_____ ____

_____ ____

_____ ____

_____ ____

_____ ____

_____ ____

NOTES

_____

_____

_____

_____

_____

_____

_____

DAY 3

FOOD TRACKING

DESCRIPTION	CALORIE/ FAT/CARB
_____	_____
_____	_____
_____	_____
_____	_____
_____	_____
_____	_____
_____	_____
_____	_____
_____	_____
_____	_____
_____	_____
_____	_____
_____	_____
_____	_____
_____	_____
_____	_____
_____	_____
_____	_____

TOTALS _____

GLASSES OF WATER CHECK-LIST

☐　☐　☐　☐

☐　☐　☐　☐

DAILY EXERCISES (SEE EXERCISE LIST)

DESCRIPTION	TIME
_____	____
_____	____
_____	____
_____	____
_____	____
_____	____

NOTES

_____

_____

_____

_____

_____

_____

_____

DAY 4

FOOD TRACKING

DESCRIPTION   **CALORIE/**
                        FAT/CARB

_____   _____

_____   _____

_____   _____

_____   _____

_____   _____

_____   _____

_____   _____

_____   _____

_____   _____

_____   _____

_____   _____

_____   _____

_____   _____

_____   _____

_____   _____

_____   _____

_____   _____

_____   _____

TOTALS   _____

GLASSES OF WATER CHECK-LIST

☐   ☐   ☐   ☐

☐   ☐   ☐   ☐

DAILY EXERCISES (SEE EXERCISE LIST)

DESCRIPTION   **TIME**

_____   _____

_____   _____

_____   _____

_____   _____

_____   _____

_____   _____

NOTES

_____

_____

_____

_____

_____

_____

_____

DAY 5

FOOD TRACKING

DESCRIPTION   CALORIE/
                      FAT/CARB

_____ _____

_____ _____

_____ _____

_____ _____

_____ _____

_____ _____

_____ _____

_____ _____

_____ _____

_____ _____

_____ _____

_____ _____

_____ _____

_____ _____

_____ _____

_____ _____

_____ _____

TOTALS   _____

GLASSES OF WATER CHECK-LIST

☐   ☐   ☐   ☐

☐   ☐   ☐   ☐

DAILY EXERCISES (SEE EXERCISE LIST)

DESCRIPTION   TIME

_____ _____

_____ _____

_____ _____

_____ _____

_____ _____

_____ _____

NOTES

_____

_____

_____

_____

_____

_____

_____

_____

43

DAY 6

FOOD TRACKING

DESCRIPTION	CALORIE/ FAT/CARB
_____	_____
_____	_____
_____	_____
_____	_____
_____	_____
_____	_____
_____	_____
_____	_____
_____	_____
_____	_____
_____	_____
_____	_____
_____	_____
_____	_____
_____	_____
_____	_____
_____	_____

TOTALS _____

GLASSES OF WATER CHECK-LIST

☐ ☐ ☐ ☐
☐ ☐ ☐ ☐

DAILY EXERCISES (SEE EXERCISE LIST)

DESCRIPTION	TIME
_____	_____
_____	_____
_____	_____
_____	_____
_____	_____
_____	_____

NOTES

_____
_____
_____
_____
_____
_____
_____

DAY 7

FOOD TRACKING

DESCRIPTION	CALORIE/ FAT/CARB
_____	_____
_____	_____
_____	_____
_____	_____
_____	_____
_____	_____
_____	_____
_____	_____
_____	_____
_____	_____
_____	_____
_____	_____
_____	_____
_____	_____
_____	_____
_____	_____
_____	_____

TOTALS _____

GLASSES OF WATER CHECK-LIST

☐ ☐ ☐ ☐

☐ ☐ ☐ ☐

DAILY EXERCISES (SEE EXERCISE LIST)

DESCRIPTION	TIME
_____	____
_____	____
_____	____
_____	____
_____	____
_____	____

NOTES

_____

_____

_____

_____

_____

_____

_____

45

WEEKLY TOTALS

	CALORIES FAT OR CARBS	WATER	EXERCISE TIME
DAY 1	_____	_____	_____
DAY 2	_____	_____	_____
DAY 3	_____	_____	_____
DAY 4	_____	_____	_____
DAY 5	_____	_____	_____
DAY 6	_____	_____	_____
DAY 7	_____	_____	_____
TOTALS	_____	_____	_____

DAY 1

FOOD TRACKING

DESCRIPTION   **CALORIE/**
                                   FAT/CARB

_____   _____

_____   _____

_____   _____

_____   _____

_____   _____

_____   _____

_____   _____

_____   _____

_____   _____

_____   _____

_____   _____

_____   _____

_____   _____

_____   _____

_____   _____

_____   _____

_____   _____

TOTALS   _____

GLASSES OF WATER CHECK-LIST

☐   ☐   ☐   ☐

☐   ☐   ☐   ☐

DAILY EXERCISES (SEE EXERCISE LIST)

DESCRIPTION   **TIME**

_____   ____

_____   ____

_____   ____

_____   ____

_____   ____

_____   ____

NOTES

_____

_____

_____

_____

_____

_____

_____

DAY 2

FOOD TRACKING

DESCRIPTION	CALORIE/ FAT/CARB
_____	_____
_____	_____
_____	_____
_____	_____
_____	_____
_____	_____
_____	_____
_____	_____
_____	_____
_____	_____
_____	_____
_____	_____
_____	_____
_____	_____
_____	_____
_____	_____
_____	_____
_____	_____
TOTALS	_____

GLASSES OF WATER CHECK-LIST

☐　☐　☐　☐

☐　☐　☐　☐

DAILY EXERCISES (SEE EXERCISE LIST)

DESCRIPTION	TIME
_____	_____
_____	_____
_____	_____
_____	_____
_____	_____
_____	_____

NOTES

_____

_____

_____

_____

_____

_____

_____

DAY 3

FOOD TRACKING

DESCRIPTION   CALORIE/
                               FAT/CARB

_____   _____

_____   _____

_____   _____

_____   _____

_____   _____

_____   _____

_____   _____

_____   _____

_____   _____

_____   _____

_____   _____

_____   _____

_____   _____

_____   _____

_____   _____

_____   _____

_____   _____

TOTALS   _____

GLASSES OF WATER CHECK-LIST

☐   ☐   ☐   ☐

☐   ☐   ☐   ☐

DAILY EXERCISES (SEE EXERCISE LIST)

DESCRIPTION   TIME

_____   _____

_____   _____

_____   _____

_____   _____

_____   _____

_____   _____

NOTES

_____

_____

_____

_____

_____

_____

_____

DAY 4

FOOD TRACKING

DESCRIPTION   **CALORIE/**
                              FAT/CARB

_____   _____

_____   _____

_____   _____

_____   _____

_____   _____

_____   _____

_____   _____

_____   _____

_____   _____

_____   _____

_____   _____

_____   _____

_____   _____

_____   _____

_____   _____

_____   _____

TOTALS   _____

GLASSES OF WATER CHECK-LIST

☐   ☐   ☐   ☐

☐   ☐   ☐   ☐

DAILY EXERCISES (SEE EXERCISE LIST)

DESCRIPTION   **TIME**

_____   _____

_____   _____

_____   _____

_____   _____

_____   _____

_____   _____

NOTES

_____

_____

_____

_____

_____

_____

_____

50

DAY 5

FOOD TRACKING

DESCRIPTION	CALORIE/ FAT/CARB
_____	_____
_____	_____
_____	_____
_____	_____
_____	_____
_____	_____
_____	_____
_____	_____
_____	_____
_____	_____
_____	_____
_____	_____
_____	_____
_____	_____
_____	_____
_____	_____
_____	_____

GLASSES OF WATER CHECK-LIST

☐ ☐ ☐ ☐
☐ ☐ ☐ ☐

DAILY EXERCISES (SEE EXERCISE LIST)

DESCRIPTION	TIME
_____	_____
_____	_____
_____	_____
_____	_____
_____	_____
_____	_____

NOTES

_____
_____
_____
_____
_____
_____
_____

TOTALS _____

DAY 6

FOOD TRACKING

DESCRIPTION	CALORIE/ FAT/CARB
_____	_____
_____	_____
_____	_____
_____	_____
_____	_____
_____	_____
_____	_____
_____	_____
_____	_____
_____	_____
_____	_____
_____	_____
_____	_____
_____	_____
_____	_____
_____	_____

GLASSES OF WATER CHECK-LIST

☐ ☐ ☐ ☐

☐ ☐ ☐ ☐

DAILY EXERCISES (SEE EXERCISE LIST)

DESCRIPTION	TIME
_____	_____
_____	_____
_____	_____
_____	_____
_____	_____
_____	_____

NOTES

_____

_____

_____

_____

_____

_____

_____

TOTALS _____

DAY 7

FOOD TRACKING

DESCRIPTION   **CALORIE/ FAT/CARB**

_____ _____

_____ _____

_____ _____

_____ _____

_____ _____

_____ _____

_____ _____

_____ _____

_____ _____

_____ _____

_____ _____

_____ _____

_____ _____

_____ _____

_____ _____

_____ _____

_____ _____

_____ _____

TOTALS   _____

GLASSES OF WATER CHECK-LIST

☐ ☐ ☐ ☐

☐ ☐ ☐ ☐

DAILY EXERCISES (SEE EXERCISE LIST)

DESCRIPTION   **TIME**

_____ ____

_____ ____

_____ ____

_____ ____

_____ ____

_____ ____

NOTES

_____

_____

_____

_____

_____

_____

_____

WEEKLY TOTALS

	CALORIES FAT OR CARBS	WATER	EXERCISE TIME
DAY 1	_____	_____	_____
DAY 2	_____	_____	_____
DAY 3	_____	_____	_____
DAY 4	_____	_____	_____
DAY 5	_____	_____	_____
DAY 6	_____	_____	_____
DAY 7	_____	_____	_____
TOTALS	_____	_____	_____

DAY 1

FOOD TRACKING

DESCRIPTION   CALORIE/
                            FAT/CARB

_____ _____

_____ _____

_____ _____

_____ _____

_____ _____

_____ _____

_____ _____

_____ _____

_____ _____

_____ _____

_____ _____

_____ _____

_____ _____

_____ _____

_____ _____

_____ _____

_____ _____

TOTALS   _____

GLASSES OF WATER CHECK-LIST

☐   ☐   ☐   ☐

☐   ☐   ☐   ☐

DAILY EXERCISES (SEE EXERCISE LIST)

DESCRIPTION   TIME

_____ _____

_____ _____

_____ _____

_____ _____

_____ _____

_____ _____

NOTES

_____

_____

_____

_____

_____

_____

_____

DAY 2

FOOD TRACKING

DESCRIPTION	CALORIE/FAT/CARB
_____	_____
_____	_____
_____	_____
_____	_____
_____	_____
_____	_____
_____	_____
_____	_____
_____	_____
_____	_____
_____	_____
_____	_____
_____	_____
_____	_____
_____	_____
_____	_____

TOTALS _____

GLASSES OF WATER CHECK-LIST

☐ ☐ ☐ ☐
☐ ☐ ☐ ☐

DAILY EXERCISES (SEE EXERCISE LIST)

DESCRIPTION	TIME
_____	_____
_____	_____
_____	_____
_____	_____
_____	_____
_____	_____

NOTES

_____
_____
_____
_____
_____
_____
_____

DAY 3

FOOD TRACKING

DESCRIPTION	CALORIE/ FAT/CARB
_____	_____
_____	_____
_____	_____
_____	_____
_____	_____
_____	_____
_____	_____
_____	_____
_____	_____
_____	_____
_____	_____
_____	_____
_____	_____
_____	_____
_____	_____
_____	_____

TOTALS _____

GLASSES OF WATER CHECK-LIST

☐ ☐ ☐ ☐

☐ ☐ ☐ ☐

DAILY EXERCISES (SEE EXERCISE LIST)

DESCRIPTION	TIME
_____	_____
_____	_____
_____	_____
_____	_____
_____	_____
_____	_____

NOTES

_____

_____

_____

_____

_____

_____

_____

_____

DAY 4

FOOD TRACKING

DESCRIPTION   CALORIE/
                        FAT/CARB

_____ _____

_____ _____

_____ _____

_____ _____

_____ _____

_____ _____

_____ _____

_____ _____

_____ _____

_____ _____

_____ _____

_____ _____

_____ _____

_____ _____

_____ _____

_____ _____

_____ _____

TOTALS _____

GLASSES OF WATER CHECK-LIST

☐   ☐   ☐   ☐

☐   ☐   ☐   ☐

DAILY EXERCISES (SEE EXERCISE LIST)

DESCRIPTION   TIME

_____ _____

_____ _____

_____ _____

_____ _____

_____ _____

_____ _____

NOTES

_____

_____

_____

_____

_____

_____

_____

DAY 5

FOOD TRACKING

DESCRIPTION   CALORIE/
                       FAT/CARB

_____ _____

_____ _____

_____ _____

_____ _____

_____ _____

_____ _____

_____ _____

_____ _____

_____ _____

_____ _____

_____ _____

_____ _____

_____ _____

_____ _____

_____ _____

_____ _____

TOTALS   _____

GLASSES OF WATER CHECK-LIST

☐   ☐   ☐   ☐

☐   ☐   ☐   ☐

DAILY EXERCISES (SEE EXERCISE LIST)

DESCRIPTION   TIME

_____ ____

_____ ____

_____ ____

_____ ____

_____ ____

_____ ____

NOTES

_____

_____

_____

_____

_____

_____

_____

DAY 6

FOOD TRACKING

DESCRIPTION   CALORIE/
                             FAT/CARB

_____   _____

_____   _____

_____   _____

_____   _____

_____   _____

_____   _____

_____   _____

_____   _____

_____   _____

_____   _____

_____   _____

_____   _____

_____   _____

_____   _____

TOTALS   _____

GLASSES OF WATER CHECK-LIST

☐   ☐   ☐   ☐

☐   ☐   ☐   ☐

DAILY EXERCISES (SEE EXERCISE LIST)

DESCRIPTION   TIME

_____   _____

_____   _____

_____   _____

_____   _____

_____   _____

_____   _____

NOTES

_____

_____

_____

_____

_____

_____

_____

DAY 7

FOOD TRACKING

DESCRIPTION	CALORIE/ FAT/CARB
_____	_____
_____	_____
_____	_____
_____	_____
_____	_____
_____	_____
_____	_____
_____	_____
_____	_____
_____	_____
_____	_____
_____	_____
_____	_____
_____	_____
_____	_____
_____	_____
_____	_____

TOTALS   _____

GLASSES OF WATER CHECK-LIST

☐ ☐ ☐ ☐

☐ ☐ ☐ ☐

DAILY EXERCISES (SEE EXERCISE LIST)

DESCRIPTION	TIME
_____	____
_____	____
_____	____
_____	____
_____	____
_____	____

NOTES

_____

_____

_____

_____

_____

_____

_____

WEEKLY TOTALS

	CALORIES FAT OR CARBS	WATER	EXERCISE TIME
DAY 1	_____	_____	_____
DAY 2	_____	_____	_____
DAY 3	_____	_____	_____
DAY 4	_____	_____	_____
DAY 5	_____	_____	_____
DAY 6	_____	_____	_____
DAY 7	_____	_____	_____
TOTALS	_____	_____	_____

DAY 1

FOOD TRACKING

DESCRIPTION	CALORIE/ FAT/CARB
_____	_____
_____	_____
_____	_____
_____	_____
_____	_____
_____	_____
_____	_____
_____	_____
_____	_____
_____	_____
_____	_____
_____	_____
_____	_____
_____	_____
_____	_____
_____	_____

TOTALS _____

GLASSES OF WATER CHECK-LIST

☐ ☐ ☐ ☐

☐ ☐ ☐ ☐

DAILY EXERCISES (SEE EXERCISE LIST)

DESCRIPTION	TIME
_____	_____
_____	_____
_____	_____
_____	_____
_____	_____
_____	_____

NOTES

_____

_____

_____

_____

_____

_____

_____

DAY 2

FOOD TRACKING

DESCRIPTION	CALORIE/ FAT/CARB
_____	_____
_____	_____
_____	_____
_____	_____
_____	_____
_____	_____
_____	_____
_____	_____
_____	_____
_____	_____
_____	_____
_____	_____
_____	_____
_____	_____
_____	_____
_____	_____
_____	_____

TOTALS _____

GLASSES OF WATER CHECK-LIST

☐ ☐ ☐ ☐

☐ ☐ ☐ ☐

DAILY EXERCISES (SEE EXERCISE LIST)

DESCRIPTION	TIME
_____	____
_____	____
_____	____
_____	____
_____	____
_____	____

NOTES

_____

_____

_____

_____

_____

_____

_____

DAY 3

FOOD TRACKING

DESCRIPTION	CALORIE/ FAT/CARB
_____	_____
_____	_____
_____	_____
_____	_____
_____	_____
_____	_____
_____	_____
_____	_____
_____	_____
_____	_____
_____	_____
_____	_____
_____	_____
_____	_____
_____	_____

TOTALS _____

GLASSES OF WATER CHECK-LIST

☐ ☐ ☐ ☐

☐ ☐ ☐ ☐

DAILY EXERCISES (SEE EXERCISE LIST)

DESCRIPTION	TIME
_____	_____
_____	_____
_____	_____
_____	_____
_____	_____
_____	_____

NOTES

_____

_____

_____

_____

_____

_____

_____

DAY 4

FOOD TRACKING

DESCRIPTION	CALORIE/ FAT/CARB
_____	_____
_____	_____
_____	_____
_____	_____
_____	_____
_____	_____
_____	_____
_____	_____
_____	_____
_____	_____
_____	_____
_____	_____
_____	_____
_____	_____
_____	_____

TOTALS _____

GLASSES OF WATER CHECK-LIST

☐ ☐ ☐ ☐

☐ ☐ ☐ ☐

DAILY EXERCISES (SEE EXERCISE LIST)

DESCRIPTION	TIME
_____	_____
_____	_____
_____	_____
_____	_____
_____	_____
_____	_____

NOTES

_____

_____

_____

_____

_____

_____

_____

DAY 5

FOOD TRACKING

DESCRIPTION   **CALORIE/**
                        FAT/CARB

_____ _____

_____ _____

_____ _____

_____ _____

_____ _____

_____ _____

_____ _____

_____ _____

_____ _____

_____ _____

_____ _____

_____ _____

_____ _____

_____ _____

_____ _____

_____ _____

_____ _____

_____ _____

TOTALS   _____

GLASSES OF WATER CHECK-LIST

☐   ☐   ☐   ☐

☐   ☐   ☐   ☐

DAILY EXERCISES (SEE EXERCISE LIST)

DESCRIPTION   **TIME**

_____   _____

_____   _____

_____   _____

_____   _____

_____   _____

_____   _____

NOTES

_____

_____

_____

_____

_____

_____

DAY 6

FOOD TRACKING

DESCRIPTION	CALORIE/ FAT/CARB
_____	_____
_____	_____
_____	_____
_____	_____
_____	_____
_____	_____
_____	_____
_____	_____
_____	_____
_____	_____
_____	_____
_____	_____
_____	_____
_____	_____
_____	_____

TOTALS _____

GLASSES OF WATER CHECK-LIST

☐ ☐ ☐ ☐

☐ ☐ ☐ ☐

DAILY EXERCISES (SEE EXERCISE LIST)

DESCRIPTION	TIME
_____	_____
_____	_____
_____	_____
_____	_____
_____	_____
_____	_____

NOTES

_____

_____

_____

_____

_____

_____

_____

DAY 7

FOOD TRACKING

DESCRIPTION	CALORIE/ FAT/CARB
_____	_____
_____	_____
_____	_____
_____	_____
_____	_____
_____	_____
_____	_____
_____	_____
_____	_____
_____	_____
_____	_____
_____	_____
_____	_____
_____	_____
_____	_____
_____	_____
_____	_____

TOTALS _____

GLASSES OF WATER CHECK-LIST

☐ ☐ ☐ ☐

☐ ☐ ☐ ☐

DAILY EXERCISES (SEE EXERCISE LIST)

DESCRIPTION	TIME
_____	_____
_____	_____
_____	_____
_____	_____
_____	_____
_____	_____

NOTES

_____

_____

_____

_____

_____

_____

_____

WEEKLY TOTALS

	CALORIES FAT OR CARBS	WATER	EXERCISE TIME
DAY 1	_____	_____	_____
DAY 2	_____	_____	_____
DAY 3	_____	_____	_____
DAY 4	_____	_____	_____
DAY 5	_____	_____	_____
DAY 6	_____	_____	_____
DAY 7	_____	_____	_____
TOTALS	_____	_____	_____

DAY 1

FOOD TRACKING

DESCRIPTION

CALORIE/
FAT/CARB

_____ _____

_____ _____

_____ _____

_____ _____

_____ _____

_____ _____

_____ _____

_____ _____

_____ _____

_____ _____

_____ _____

_____ _____

_____ _____

_____ _____

_____ _____

_____ _____

_____ _____

TOTALS _____

GLASSES OF WATER CHECK-LIST

☐ ☐ ☐ ☐

☐ ☐ ☐ ☐

DAILY EXERCISES (SEE EXERCISE LIST)

DESCRIPTION   TIME

_____ _____

_____ _____

_____ _____

_____ _____

_____ _____

_____ _____

NOTES

_____

_____

_____

_____

_____

_____

_____

DAY 2

FOOD TRACKING

DESCRIPTION   **CALORIE/ FAT/CARB**

_____   _____

_____   _____

_____   _____

_____   _____

_____   _____

_____   _____

_____   _____

_____   _____

_____   _____

_____   _____

_____   _____

_____   _____

_____   _____

_____   _____

_____   _____

_____   _____

TOTALS   _____

GLASSES OF WATER CHECK-LIST

☐   ☐   ☐   ☐

☐   ☐   ☐   ☐

DAILY EXERCISES (SEE EXERCISE LIST)

DESCRIPTION   **TIME**

_____   _____

_____   _____

_____   _____

_____   _____

_____   _____

_____   _____

NOTES

_____

_____

_____

_____

_____

_____

_____

DAY 3

FOOD TRACKING

DESCRIPTION	CALORIE/ FAT/CARB
_____	_____
_____	_____
_____	_____
_____	_____
_____	_____
_____	_____
_____	_____
_____	_____
_____	_____
_____	_____
_____	_____
_____	_____
_____	_____
_____	_____
_____	_____
_____	_____
_____	_____
_____	_____

TOTALS _____

GLASSES OF WATER CHECK-LIST

☐ ☐ ☐ ☐

☐ ☐ ☐ ☐

DAILY EXERCISES (SEE EXERCISE LIST)

DESCRIPTION	TIME
_____	____
_____	____
_____	____
_____	____
_____	____
_____	____

NOTES

_____

_____

_____

_____

_____

_____

_____

DAY 4

FOOD TRACKING

DESCRIPTION	CALORIE/ FAT/CARB
_____	_____
_____	_____
_____	_____
_____	_____
_____	_____
_____	_____
_____	_____
_____	_____
_____	_____
_____	_____
_____	_____
_____	_____
_____	_____
_____	_____
_____	_____
_____	_____
_____	_____

TOTALS _____

GLASSES OF WATER CHECK-LIST

☐ ☐ ☐ ☐

☐ ☐ ☐ ☐

DAILY EXERCISES (SEE EXERCISE LIST)

DESCRIPTION	TIME
_____	_____
_____	_____
_____	_____
_____	_____
_____	_____
_____	_____

NOTES

_____

_____

_____

_____

_____

_____

_____

DAY 5

FOOD TRACKING

DESCRIPTION   CALORIE/
                    FAT/CARB

_____   _____

_____   _____

_____   _____

_____   _____

_____   _____

_____   _____

_____   _____

_____   _____

_____   _____

_____   _____

_____   _____

_____   _____

_____   _____

_____   _____

_____   _____

_____   _____

_____   _____

TOTALS   _____

GLASSES OF WATER CHECK-LIST

☐   ☐   ☐   ☐

☐   ☐   ☐   ☐

DAILY EXERCISES (SEE EXERCISE LIST)

DESCRIPTION   TIME

_____   ____

_____   ____

_____   ____

_____   ____

_____   ____

_____   ____

NOTES

_____

_____

_____

_____

_____

_____

_____

DAY 6

FOOD TRACKING

DESCRIPTION	CALORIE/ FAT/CARB
_____	_____
_____	_____
_____	_____
_____	_____
_____	_____
_____	_____
_____	_____
_____	_____
_____	_____
_____	_____
_____	_____
_____	_____
_____	_____
_____	_____
_____	_____

TOTALS _____

GLASSES OF WATER CHECK-LIST

☐ ☐ ☐ ☐

☐ ☐ ☐ ☐

DAILY EXERCISES (SEE EXERCISE LIST)

DESCRIPTION	TIME
_____	____
_____	____
_____	____
_____	____
_____	____
_____	____

NOTES

_____

_____

_____

_____

_____

_____

_____

DAY 7

FOOD TRACKING

DESCRIPTION	CALORIE/ FAT/CARB
_____	_____
_____	_____
_____	_____
_____	_____
_____	_____
_____	_____
_____	_____
_____	_____
_____	_____
_____	_____
_____	_____
_____	_____
_____	_____
_____	_____
_____	_____
_____	_____

GLASSES OF WATER CHECK-LIST

☐ ☐ ☐ ☐

☐ ☐ ☐ ☐

DAILY EXERCISES (SEE EXERCISE LIST)

DESCRIPTION	TIME
_____	_____
_____	_____
_____	_____
_____	_____
_____	_____
_____	_____

NOTES

_____

_____

_____

_____

_____

_____

_____

TOTALS _____

WEEKLY TOTALS

	CALORIES FAT OR CARBS	WATER	EXERCISE TIME
DAY 1	_____	_____	_____
DAY 2	_____	_____	_____
DAY 3	_____	_____	_____
DAY 4	_____	_____	_____
DAY 5	_____	_____	_____
DAY 6	_____	_____	_____
DAY 7	_____	_____	_____
TOTALS	_____	_____	_____

DAY 1

FOOD TRACKING

DESCRIPTION	CALORIE/ FAT/CARB
_____	_____
_____	_____
_____	_____
_____	_____
_____	_____
_____	_____
_____	_____
_____	_____
_____	_____
_____	_____
_____	_____
_____	_____
_____	_____
_____	_____
_____	_____
_____	_____

TOTALS _____

GLASSES OF WATER CHECK-LIST

☐ ☐ ☐ ☐

☐ ☐ ☐ ☐

DAILY EXERCISES (SEE EXERCISE LIST)

DESCRIPTION	TIME
_____	____
_____	____
_____	____
_____	____
_____	____
_____	____

NOTES

_____

_____

_____

_____

_____

_____

_____

DAY 2

FOOD TRACKING

DESCRIPTION	CALORIE/ FAT/CARB
_____	_____
_____	_____
_____	_____
_____	_____
_____	_____
_____	_____
_____	_____
_____	_____
_____	_____
_____	_____
_____	_____
_____	_____
_____	_____
_____	_____
_____	_____
_____	_____

TOTALS _____

GLASSES OF WATER CHECK-LIST

☐   ☐   ☐   ☐

☐   ☐   ☐   ☐

DAILY EXERCISES (SEE EXERCISE LIST)

DESCRIPTION	TIME
_____	_____
_____	_____
_____	_____
_____	_____
_____	_____
_____	_____

NOTES

_____

_____

_____

_____

_____

_____

_____

DAY 3

FOOD TRACKING

DESCRIPTION	CALORIE/ FAT/CARB
_____	_____
_____	_____
_____	_____
_____	_____
_____	_____
_____	_____
_____	_____
_____	_____
_____	_____
_____	_____
_____	_____
_____	_____
_____	_____
_____	_____
_____	_____
_____	_____
_____	_____

GLASSES OF WATER CHECK-LIST

☐ ☐ ☐ ☐

☐ ☐ ☐ ☐

DAILY EXERCISES (SEE EXERCISE LIST)

DESCRIPTION	TIME
_____	_____
_____	_____
_____	_____
_____	_____
_____	_____
_____	_____

NOTES

_____

_____

_____

_____

_____

_____

_____

TOTALS _____

DAY 4

FOOD TRACKING

DESCRIPTION	CALORIE/ FAT/CARB
_____	_____
_____	_____
_____	_____
_____	_____
_____	_____
_____	_____
_____	_____
_____	_____
_____	_____
_____	_____
_____	_____
_____	_____
_____	_____
_____	_____
_____	_____
_____	_____
_____	_____
_____	_____
TOTALS	_____

GLASSES OF WATER CHECK-LIST

☐ ☐ ☐ ☐

☐ ☐ ☐ ☐

DAILY EXERCISES (SEE EXERCISE LIST)

DESCRIPTION	TIME
_____	_____
_____	_____
_____	_____
_____	_____
_____	_____
_____	_____

NOTES

_____

_____

_____

_____

_____

_____

_____

DAY 5

FOOD TRACKING

GLASSES OF WATER CHECK-LIST

DESCRIPTION   CALORIE/
                              FAT/CARB

☐   ☐   ☐   ☐

☐   ☐   ☐   ☐

DAILY EXERCISES (SEE EXERCISE LIST)

DESCRIPTION   TIME

NOTES

TOTALS _____

83

DAY 6

FOOD TRACKING

DESCRIPTION	CALORIE/ FAT/CARB
_____	_____
_____	_____
_____	_____
_____	_____
_____	_____
_____	_____
_____	_____
_____	_____
_____	_____
_____	_____
_____	_____
_____	_____
_____	_____
_____	_____
_____	_____

TOTALS _____

GLASSES OF WATER CHECK-LIST

☐ ☐ ☐ ☐

☐ ☐ ☐ ☐

DAILY EXERCISES (SEE EXERCISE LIST)

DESCRIPTION	TIME
_____	_____
_____	_____
_____	_____
_____	_____
_____	_____
_____	_____

NOTES

_____

_____

_____

_____

_____

_____

_____

DAY 7

FOOD TRACKING

GLASSES OF WATER CHECK-LIST

DESCRIPTION

CALORIE/
FAT/CARB

☐ ☐ ☐ ☐

☐ ☐ ☐ ☐

_____ _____

_____ _____

_____ _____

_____ _____

_____ _____

DAILY EXERCISES (SEE EXERCISE LIST)

DESCRIPTION

TIME

_____ _____

_____ _____

_____ _____

_____ _____

_____ _____

_____ _____

_____ _____

_____ _____

_____ _____

_____ _____

_____ _____

NOTES

_____ _____

_____ _____

_____

_____ _____

_____

_____ _____

_____

_____ _____

_____

_____ _____

_____

_____

_____

TOTALS _____

85

WEEKLY TOTALS

	CALORIES FAT OR CARBS	WATER	EXERCISE TIME
DAY 1	_____	_____	_____
DAY 2	_____	_____	_____
DAY 3	_____	_____	_____
DAY 4	_____	_____	_____
DAY 5	_____	_____	_____
DAY 6	_____	_____	_____
DAY 7	_____	_____	_____
TOTALS	_____	_____	_____

DAY 1

FOOD TRACKING

DESCRIPTION	CALORIE/ FAT/CARB
_____	_____
_____	_____
_____	_____
_____	_____
_____	_____
_____	_____
_____	_____
_____	_____
_____	_____
_____	_____
_____	_____
_____	_____
_____	_____
_____	_____
_____	_____
_____	_____
_____	_____

TOTALS _____

GLASSES OF WATER CHECK-LIST

☐ ☐ ☐ ☐

☐ ☐ ☐ ☐

DAILY EXERCISES (SEE EXERCISE LIST)

DESCRIPTION	TIME
_____	____
_____	____
_____	____
_____	____
_____	____
_____	____

NOTES

_____

_____

_____

_____

_____

_____

_____

DAY 2

FOOD TRACKING

DESCRIPTION　　　**CALORIE/ FAT/CARB**

_____　_____

_____　_____

_____　_____

_____　_____

_____　_____

_____　_____

_____　_____

_____　_____

_____　_____

_____　_____

_____　_____

_____　_____

_____　_____

_____　_____

_____　_____

TOTALS　　　　　　　_____

GLASSES OF WATER CHECK-LIST

☐　　☐　　☐　　☐

☐　　☐　　☐　　☐

DAILY EXERCISES (SEE EXERCISE LIST)

DESCRIPTION　　　　　　**TIME**

_____　_____

_____　_____

_____　_____

_____　_____

_____　_____

_____　_____

NOTES

_____

_____

_____

_____

_____

_____

_____

DAY 3

FOOD TRACKING

DESCRIPTION	CALORIE/ FAT/CARB
_____	_____
_____	_____
_____	_____
_____	_____
_____	_____
_____	_____
_____	_____
_____	_____
_____	_____
_____	_____
_____	_____
_____	_____
_____	_____
_____	_____
_____	_____
_____	_____
_____	_____

TOTALS _____

GLASSES OF WATER CHECK-LIST

☐ ☐ ☐ ☐

☐ ☐ ☐ ☐

DAILY EXERCISES (SEE EXERCISE LIST)

DESCRIPTION	TIME
_____	____
_____	____
_____	____
_____	____
_____	____
_____	____

NOTES

_____

_____

_____

_____

_____

_____

_____

DAY 4

FOOD TRACKING

DESCRIPTION	CALORIE/ FAT/CARB
_____	_____
_____	_____
_____	_____
_____	_____
_____	_____
_____	_____
_____	_____
_____	_____
_____	_____
_____	_____
_____	_____
_____	_____
_____	_____
_____	_____
_____	_____

TOTALS _____

GLASSES OF WATER CHECK-LIST

☐ ☐ ☐ ☐

☐ ☐ ☐ ☐

DAILY EXERCISES (SEE EXERCISE LIST)

DESCRIPTION	TIME
_____	___
_____	___
_____	___
_____	___
_____	___
_____	___

NOTES

_____

_____

_____

_____

_____

_____

_____

DAY 5

FOOD TRACKING

DESCRIPTION   **CALORIE/**
                            FAT/CARB

_____ _____

_____ _____

_____ _____

_____ _____

_____ _____

_____ _____

_____ _____

_____ _____

_____ _____

_____ _____

_____ _____

_____ _____

_____ _____

_____ _____

_____ _____

_____ _____

GLASSES OF WATER CHECK-LIST

☐ ☐ ☐ ☐

☐ ☐ ☐ ☐

DAILY EXERCISES (SEE EXERCISE LIST)

DESCRIPTION   **TIME**

_____ ____

_____ ____

_____ ____

_____ ____

_____ ____

_____ ____

NOTES

_____

_____

_____

_____

_____

_____

_____

TOTALS   _____

DAY 6

FOOD TRACKING

DESCRIPTION   CALORIE/
                            FAT/CARB

_____   _____

_____   _____

_____   _____

_____   _____

_____   _____

_____   _____

_____   _____

_____   _____

_____   _____

_____   _____

_____   _____

_____   _____

_____   _____

_____   _____

_____   _____

_____   _____

_____   _____

TOTALS   _____

GLASSES OF WATER CHECK-LIST

☐   ☐   ☐   ☐

☐   ☐   ☐   ☐

DAILY EXERCISES (SEE EXERCISE LIST)

DESCRIPTION   TIME

_____   _____

_____   _____

_____   _____

_____   _____

_____   _____

_____   _____

NOTES

_____

_____

_____

_____

_____

_____

DAY 7

FOOD TRACKING

DESCRIPTION	CALORIE/ FAT/CARB
_____	_____
_____	_____
_____	_____
_____	_____
_____	_____
_____	_____
_____	_____
_____	_____
_____	_____
_____	_____
_____	_____
_____	_____
_____	_____
_____	_____
_____	_____

TOTALS _____

GLASSES OF WATER CHECK-LIST

☐ ☐ ☐ ☐

☐ ☐ ☐ ☐

DAILY EXERCISES (SEE EXERCISE LIST)

DESCRIPTION	TIME
_____	____
_____	____
_____	____
_____	____
_____	____
_____	____

NOTES

_____

_____

_____

_____

_____

_____

_____

WEEKLY TOTALS

	CALORIES FAT OR CARBS	WATER	EXERCISE TIME
DAY 1	_____	_____	_____
DAY 2	_____	_____	_____
DAY 3	_____	_____	_____
DAY 4	_____	_____	_____
DAY 5	_____	_____	_____
DAY 6	_____	_____	_____
DAY 7	_____	_____	_____
TOTALS	_____	_____	_____

DAY 1

FOOD TRACKING

DESCRIPTION   **CALORIE/**
                              FAT/CARB

_____   _____

_____   _____

_____   _____

_____   _____

_____   _____

_____   _____

_____   _____

_____   _____

_____   _____

_____   _____

_____   _____

_____   _____

_____   _____

_____   _____

_____   _____

TOTALS   _____

GLASSES OF WATER CHECK-LIST

☐   ☐   ☐   ☐

☐   ☐   ☐   ☐

DAILY EXERCISES (SEE EXERCISE LIST)

DESCRIPTION   **TIME**

_____   _____

_____   _____

_____   _____

_____   _____

_____   _____

_____   _____

NOTES

_____

_____

_____

_____

_____

_____

_____

DAY 2

FOOD TRACKING

DESCRIPTION	CALORIE/ FAT/CARB
_____	_____
_____	_____
_____	_____
_____	_____
_____	_____
_____	_____
_____	_____
_____	_____
_____	_____
_____	_____
_____	_____
_____	_____
_____	_____
_____	_____
_____	_____
_____	_____

GLASSES OF WATER CHECK-LIST

☐ ☐ ☐ ☐

☐ ☐ ☐ ☐

DAILY EXERCISES (SEE EXERCISE LIST)

DESCRIPTION	TIME
_____	____
_____	____
_____	____
_____	____
_____	____
_____	____

NOTES

_____

_____

_____

_____

_____

_____

_____

TOTALS _____

DAY 3

FOOD TRACKING

DESCRIPTION	CALORIE/ FAT/CARB
_____	_____
_____	_____
_____	_____
_____	_____
_____	_____
_____	_____
_____	_____
_____	_____
_____	_____
_____	_____
_____	_____
_____	_____
_____	_____
_____	_____
_____	_____

TOTALS _____

GLASSES OF WATER CHECK-LIST

☐ ☐ ☐ ☐

☐ ☐ ☐ ☐

DAILY EXERCISES (SEE EXERCISE LIST)

DESCRIPTION	TIME
_____	_____
_____	_____
_____	_____
_____	_____
_____	_____
_____	_____

NOTES

_____

_____

_____

_____

_____

_____

_____

DAY 4

FOOD TRACKING

DESCRIPTION	CALORIE/ FAT/CARB
_____	_____
_____	_____
_____	_____
_____	_____
_____	_____
_____	_____
_____	_____
_____	_____
_____	_____
_____	_____
_____	_____
_____	_____
_____	_____
_____	_____
_____	_____
_____	_____

TOTALS _____

GLASSES OF WATER CHECK-LIST

☐ ☐ ☐ ☐

☐ ☐ ☐ ☐

DAILY EXERCISES (SEE EXERCISE LIST)

DESCRIPTION	TIME
_____	_____
_____	_____
_____	_____
_____	_____
_____	_____
_____	_____

NOTES

_____

_____

_____

_____

_____

_____

_____

DAY 5

FOOD TRACKING

DESCRIPTION	CALORIE/ FAT/CARB
_____	_____
_____	_____
_____	_____
_____	_____
_____	_____
_____	_____
_____	_____
_____	_____
_____	_____
_____	_____
_____	_____
_____	_____
_____	_____
_____	_____
_____	_____
_____	_____

TOTALS _____

GLASSES OF WATER CHECK-LIST

☐ ☐ ☐ ☐

☐ ☐ ☐ ☐

DAILY EXERCISES (SEE EXERCISE LIST)

DESCRIPTION	TIME
_____	____
_____	____
_____	____
_____	____
_____	____
_____	____

NOTES

_____

_____

_____

_____

_____

_____

_____

DAY 6

FOOD TRACKING

DESCRIPTION	CALORIE/ FAT/CARB
_____	_____
_____	_____
_____	_____
_____	_____
_____	_____
_____	_____
_____	_____
_____	_____
_____	_____
_____	_____
_____	_____
_____	_____
_____	_____
_____	_____
_____	_____

TOTALS _____

GLASSES OF WATER CHECK-LIST

☐ ☐ ☐ ☐

☐ ☐ ☐ ☐

DAILY EXERCISES (SEE EXERCISE LIST)

DESCRIPTION	TIME
_____	_____
_____	_____
_____	_____
_____	_____
_____	_____
_____	_____

NOTES

_____

_____

_____

_____

_____

_____

_____

DAY 7

FOOD TRACKING

DESCRIPTION	CALORIE/ FAT/CARB
_____	_____
_____	_____
_____	_____
_____	_____
_____	_____
_____	_____
_____	_____
_____	_____
_____	_____
_____	_____
_____	_____
_____	_____
_____	_____
_____	_____
_____	_____
_____	_____

TOTALS _____

GLASSES OF WATER CHECK-LIST

☐ ☐ ☐ ☐

☐ ☐ ☐ ☐

DAILY EXERCISES (SEE EXERCISE LIST)

DESCRIPTION	TIME
_____	_____
_____	_____
_____	_____
_____	_____
_____	_____
_____	_____

NOTES

_____

_____

_____

_____

_____

_____

_____

WEEKLY TOTALS

	CALORIES FAT OR CARBS	WATER	EXERCISE TIME
DAY 1	_____	_____	_____
DAY 2	_____	_____	_____
DAY 3	_____	_____	_____
DAY 4	_____	_____	_____
DAY 5	_____	_____	_____
DAY 6	_____	_____	_____
DAY 7	_____	_____	_____
TOTALS	_____	_____	_____

DAY 1

FOOD TRACKING

DESCRIPTION	CALORIE/ FAT/CARB
_____	_____
_____	_____
_____	_____
_____	_____
_____	_____
_____	_____
_____	_____
_____	_____
_____	_____
_____	_____
_____	_____
_____	_____
_____	_____
_____	_____
_____	_____
_____	_____

TOTALS _____

GLASSES OF WATER CHECK-LIST

☐ ☐ ☐ ☐

☐ ☐ ☐ ☐

DAILY EXERCISES (SEE EXERCISE LIST)

DESCRIPTION	TIME
_____	____
_____	____
_____	____
_____	____
_____	____
_____	____

NOTES

_____

_____

_____

_____

_____

_____

_____

DAY 2

FOOD TRACKING

DESCRIPTION	CALORIE/ FAT/CARB
_____	_____
_____	_____
_____	_____
_____	_____
_____	_____
_____	_____
_____	_____
_____	_____
_____	_____
_____	_____
_____	_____
_____	_____
_____	_____
_____	_____
_____	_____
_____	_____

TOTALS _____

GLASSES OF WATER CHECK-LIST

☐ ☐ ☐ ☐

☐ ☐ ☐ ☐

DAILY EXERCISES (SEE EXERCISE LIST)

DESCRIPTION	TIME
_____	____
_____	____
_____	____
_____	____
_____	____
_____	____

NOTES

_____

_____

_____

_____

_____

_____

_____

DAY 3

FOOD TRACKING

DESCRIPTION	CALORIE/ FAT/CARB
_____	_____
_____	_____
_____	_____
_____	_____
_____	_____
_____	_____
_____	_____
_____	_____
_____	_____
_____	_____
_____	_____
_____	_____
_____	_____
_____	_____
_____	_____
_____	_____
_____	_____
_____	_____

TOTALS _____

GLASSES OF WATER CHECK-LIST

☐   ☐   ☐   ☐

☐   ☐   ☐   ☐

DAILY EXERCISES (SEE EXERCISE LIST)

DESCRIPTION	TIME
_____	_____
_____	_____
_____	_____
_____	_____
_____	_____
_____	_____

NOTES

_____

_____

_____

_____

_____

_____

_____

DAY 4

FOOD TRACKING

DESCRIPTION	CALORIE/ FAT/CARB
_____	_____
_____	_____
_____	_____
_____	_____
_____	_____
_____	_____
_____	_____
_____	_____
_____	_____
_____	_____
_____	_____
_____	_____
_____	_____
_____	_____
_____	_____
_____	_____
_____	_____
_____	_____

TOTALS _____

GLASSES OF WATER CHECK-LIST

☐ ☐ ☐ ☐

☐ ☐ ☐ ☐

DAILY EXERCISES (SEE EXERCISE LIST)

DESCRIPTION	TIME
_____	_____
_____	_____
_____	_____
_____	_____
_____	_____
_____	_____

NOTES

_____

_____

_____

_____

_____

_____

_____

DAY 5

FOOD TRACKING

DESCRIPTION   CALORIE/
                          FAT/CARB

_____ _____

_____ _____

_____ _____

_____ _____

_____ _____

_____ _____

_____ _____

_____ _____

_____ _____

_____ _____

_____ _____

_____ _____

_____ _____

_____ _____

_____ _____

_____ _____

TOTALS   _____

GLASSES OF WATER CHECK-LIST

☐   ☐   ☐   ☐

☐   ☐   ☐   ☐

DAILY EXERCISES (SEE EXERCISE LIST)

DESCRIPTION   TIME

_____ _____

_____ _____

_____ _____

_____ _____

_____ _____

_____ _____

NOTES

_____

_____

_____

_____

_____

_____

_____

DAY 6

FOOD TRACKING

DESCRIPTION   **CALORIE/
                                 FAT/CARB**

_____   _____

_____   _____

_____   _____

_____   _____

_____   _____

_____   _____

_____   _____

_____   _____

_____   _____

_____   _____

_____   _____

_____   _____

_____   _____

_____   _____

_____   _____

TOTALS   _____

GLASSES OF WATER CHECK-LIST

☐   ☐   ☐   ☐

☐   ☐   ☐   ☐

DAILY EXERCISES (SEE EXERCISE LIST)

DESCRIPTION   **TIME**

_____   ____

_____   ____

_____   ____

_____   ____

_____   ____

_____   ____

NOTES

_____

_____

_____

_____

_____

_____

_____

DAY 7

FOOD TRACKING

DESCRIPTION	CALORIE/ FAT/CARB
_____	_____
_____	_____
_____	_____
_____	_____
_____	_____
_____	_____
_____	_____
_____	_____
_____	_____
_____	_____
_____	_____
_____	_____
_____	_____
_____	_____
_____	_____
_____	_____
_____	_____
_____	_____

TOTALS _____

GLASSES OF WATER CHECK-LIST

☐ ☐ ☐ ☐

☐ ☐ ☐ ☐

DAILY EXERCISES (SEE EXERCISE LIST)

DESCRIPTION	TIME
_____	____
_____	____
_____	____
_____	____
_____	____
_____	____

NOTES

_____

_____

_____

_____

_____

_____

_____

WEEKLY TOTALS

	CALORIES FAT OR CARBS	WATER	EXERCISE TIME
DAY 1	_____	_____	_____
DAY 2	_____	_____	_____
DAY 3	_____	_____	_____
DAY 4	_____	_____	_____
DAY 5	_____	_____	_____
DAY 6	_____	_____	_____
DAY 7	_____	_____	_____
TOTALS	_____	_____	_____

DAY 1

FOOD TRACKING

DESCRIPTION   **CALORIE/**
                          FAT/CARB

_____   _____

_____   _____

_____   _____

_____   _____

_____   _____

_____   _____

_____   _____

_____   _____

_____   _____

_____   _____

_____   _____

_____   _____

_____   _____

_____   _____

_____   _____

_____   _____

TOTALS   _____

GLASSES OF WATER CHECK-LIST

☐   ☐   ☐   ☐

☐   ☐   ☐   ☐

DAILY EXERCISES (SEE EXERCISE LIST)

DESCRIPTION   **TIME**

_____   _____

_____   _____

_____   _____

_____   _____

_____   _____

_____   _____

NOTES

_____

_____

_____

_____

_____

_____

_____

111

DAY 2

FOOD TRACKING

DESCRIPTION	CALORIE/ FAT/CARB
_____	_____
_____	_____
_____	_____
_____	_____
_____	_____
_____	_____
_____	_____
_____	_____
_____	_____
_____	_____
_____	_____
_____	_____
_____	_____
_____	_____
_____	_____
_____	_____

TOTALS _____

GLASSES OF WATER CHECK-LIST

☐ ☐ ☐ ☐
☐ ☐ ☐ ☐

DAILY EXERCISES (SEE EXERCISE LIST)

DESCRIPTION	TIME
_____	_____
_____	_____
_____	_____
_____	_____
_____	_____
_____	_____

NOTES

_____

_____

_____

_____

_____

_____

_____

DAY 3

FOOD TRACKING

DESCRIPTION	CALORIE/ FAT/CARB
_____	_____
_____	_____
_____	_____
_____	_____
_____	_____
_____	_____
_____	_____
_____	_____
_____	_____
_____	_____
_____	_____
_____	_____
_____	_____
_____	_____
_____	_____

TOTALS _____

GLASSES OF WATER CHECK-LIST

☐ ☐ ☐ ☐

☐ ☐ ☐ ☐

DAILY EXERCISES (SEE EXERCISE LIST)

DESCRIPTION	TIME
_____	_____
_____	_____
_____	_____
_____	_____
_____	_____
_____	_____

NOTES

_____

_____

_____

_____

_____

_____

_____

DAY 4

FOOD TRACKING

DESCRIPTION   **CALORIE/**
                         FAT/CARB

_____ _____

_____ _____

_____ _____

_____ _____

_____ _____

_____ _____

_____ _____

_____ _____

_____ _____

_____ _____

_____ _____

_____ _____

_____ _____

_____ _____

_____ _____

_____ _____

_____ _____

_____ _____

TOTALS   _____

GLASSES OF WATER CHECK-LIST

☐   ☐   ☐   ☐

☐   ☐   ☐   ☐

DAILY EXERCISES (SEE EXERCISE LIST)

DESCRIPTION   **TIME**

_____ _____

_____ _____

_____ _____

_____ _____

_____ _____

_____ _____

NOTES

_____

_____

_____

_____

_____

_____

_____

DAY 5

FOOD TRACKING

DESCRIPTION	CALORIE/ FAT/CARB
_____	_____
_____	_____
_____	_____
_____	_____
_____	_____
_____	_____
_____	_____
_____	_____
_____	_____
_____	_____
_____	_____
_____	_____
_____	_____
_____	_____
_____	_____
_____	_____

TOTALS _____

GLASSES OF WATER CHECK-LIST

☐ ☐ ☐ ☐

☐ ☐ ☐ ☐

DAILY EXERCISES (SEE EXERCISE LIST)

DESCRIPTION	TIME
_____	____
_____	____
_____	____
_____	____
_____	____
_____	____

NOTES

_____

_____

_____

_____

_____

_____

_____

DAY 6

FOOD TRACKING

DESCRIPTION	CALORIE/ FAT/CARB
_____	_____
_____	_____
_____	_____
_____	_____
_____	_____
_____	_____
_____	_____
_____	_____
_____	_____
_____	_____
_____	_____
_____	_____
_____	_____
_____	_____
_____	_____
_____	_____
_____	_____
_____	_____

TOTALS _____

GLASSES OF WATER CHECK-LIST

☐   ☐   ☐   ☐

☐   ☐   ☐   ☐

DAILY EXERCISES (SEE EXERCISE LIST)

DESCRIPTION	TIME
_____	_____
_____	_____
_____	_____
_____	_____
_____	_____

NOTES

_____

_____

_____

_____

_____

_____

_____

DAY 7

FOOD TRACKING

DESCRIPTION　　　　**CALORIE/**
　　　　　　　　　　　FAT/CARB

_____　_____

_____　_____

_____　_____

_____　_____

_____　_____

_____　_____

_____　_____

_____　_____

_____　_____

_____　_____

_____　_____

_____　_____

_____　_____

_____　_____

_____　_____

TOTALS　　　　　_____

GLASSES OF WATER CHECK-LIST

☐　　☐　　☐　　☐

☐　　☐　　☐　　☐

DAILY EXERCISES (SEE EXERCISE LIST)

DESCRIPTION　　　　　　　**TIME**

_____　_____

_____　_____

_____　_____

_____　_____

_____　_____

_____　_____

NOTES

_____

_____

_____

_____

_____

_____

_____

WEEKLY TOTALS

	CALORIES FAT OR CARBS	WATER	EXERCISE TIME
DAY 1	_____	_____	_____
DAY 2	_____	_____	_____
DAY 3	_____	_____	_____
DAY 4	_____	_____	_____
DAY 5	_____	_____	_____
DAY 6	_____	_____	_____
DAY 7	_____	_____	_____
TOTALS	_____	_____	_____

DAY 1

FOOD TRACKING

DESCRIPTION   **CALORIE/**
                          FAT/CARB

_____   _____

_____   _____

_____   _____

_____   _____

_____   _____

_____   _____

_____   _____

_____   _____

_____   _____

_____   _____

_____   _____

_____   _____

_____   _____

_____   _____

_____   _____

TOTALS   _____

GLASSES OF WATER CHECK-LIST

☐   ☐   ☐   ☐

☐   ☐   ☐   ☐

DAILY EXERCISES (SEE EXERCISE LIST)

DESCRIPTION   **TIME**

_____   _____

_____   _____

_____   _____

_____   _____

_____   _____

_____   _____

NOTES

_____

_____

_____

_____

_____

_____

_____

DAY 2

FOOD TRACKING

DESCRIPTION	CALORIE/ FAT/CARB
_____	_____
_____	_____
_____	_____
_____	_____
_____	_____
_____	_____
_____	_____
_____	_____
_____	_____
_____	_____
_____	_____
_____	_____
_____	_____
_____	_____
_____	_____
_____	_____
_____	_____

GLASSES OF WATER CHECK-LIST

☐ ☐ ☐ ☐

☐ ☐ ☐ ☐

DAILY EXERCISES (SEE EXERCISE LIST)

DESCRIPTION	TIME
_____	_____
_____	_____
_____	_____
_____	_____
_____	_____
_____	_____

NOTES

_____

_____

_____

_____

_____

_____

_____

TOTALS _____

DAY 3

FOOD TRACKING

DESCRIPTION
                               **CALORIE/
FAT/CARB**

_____ _____

_____ _____

_____ _____

_____ _____

_____ _____

_____ _____

_____ _____

_____ _____

_____ _____

_____ _____

_____ _____

_____ _____

_____ _____

_____ _____

_____ _____

_____ _____

TOTALS   _____

GLASSES OF WATER CHECK-LIST

☐ ☐ ☐ ☐

☐ ☐ ☐ ☐

DAILY EXERCISES (SEE EXERCISE LIST)

DESCRIPTION   **TIME**

_____ _____

_____ _____

_____ _____

_____ _____

_____ _____

_____ _____

NOTES

_____

_____

_____

_____

_____

_____

_____

121

DAY 4

FOOD TRACKING

DESCRIPTION　　　　**CALORIE/**
　　　　　　　　　　　FAT/CARB

_____　_____

_____　_____

_____　_____

_____　_____

_____　_____

_____　_____

_____　_____

_____　_____

_____　_____

_____　_____

_____　_____

_____　_____

_____　_____

_____　_____

_____　_____

_____　_____

_____　_____

TOTALS　　　　　　_____

GLASSES OF WATER CHECK-LIST

☐　　☐　　☐　　☐

☐　　☐　　☐　　☐

DAILY EXERCISES (SEE EXERCISE LIST)

DESCRIPTION　　　　　　**TIME**

_____　____

_____　____

_____　____

_____　____

_____　____

_____　____

NOTES

_____

_____

_____

_____

_____

_____

_____

DAY 5

FOOD TRACKING

DESCRIPTION   **CALORIE/
FAT/CARB**

_____ _____

_____ _____

_____ _____

_____ _____

_____ _____

_____ _____

_____ _____

_____ _____

_____ _____

_____ _____

_____ _____

_____ _____

_____ _____

_____ _____

_____ _____

_____ _____

TOTALS   _____

GLASSES OF WATER CHECK-LIST

☐ ☐ ☐ ☐

☐ ☐ ☐ ☐

DAILY EXERCISES (SEE EXERCISE LIST)

DESCRIPTION   **TIME**

_____ _____

_____ _____

_____ _____

_____ _____

_____ _____

_____ _____

NOTES

_____

_____

_____

_____

_____

_____

_____

DAY 6

FOOD TRACKING

DESCRIPTION   **CALORIE/**
                               FAT/CARB

_____   _____

_____   _____

_____   _____

_____   _____

_____   _____

_____   _____

_____   _____

_____   _____

_____   _____

_____   _____

_____   _____

_____   _____

_____   _____

_____   _____

_____   _____

TOTALS   _____

GLASSES OF WATER CHECK-LIST

☐   ☐   ☐   ☐

☐   ☐   ☐   ☐

DAILY EXERCISES (SEE EXERCISE LIST)

DESCRIPTION   **TIME**

_____   _____

_____   _____

_____   _____

_____   _____

_____   _____

_____   _____

NOTES

_____

_____

_____

_____

_____

_____

_____

DAY 7

FOOD TRACKING

GLASSES OF WATER CHECK-LIST

DESCRIPTION	CALORIE/ FAT/CARB
_____	_____
_____	_____
_____	_____
_____	_____
_____	_____
_____	_____
_____	_____
_____	_____
_____	_____
_____	_____
_____	_____
_____	_____
_____	_____
_____	_____
_____	_____
_____	_____
_____	_____

☐ ☐ ☐ ☐

☐ ☐ ☐ ☐

DAILY EXERCISES (SEE EXERCISE LIST)

DESCRIPTION	TIME
_____	____
_____	____
_____	____
_____	____
_____	____
_____	____

NOTES

_____

_____

_____

_____

_____

_____

_____

TOTALS _____

WEEKLY TOTALS

	CALORIES FAT OR CARBS	WATER	EXERCISE TIME
DAY 1	_____	_____	_____
DAY 2	_____	_____	_____
DAY 3	_____	_____	_____
DAY 4	_____	_____	_____
DAY 5	_____	_____	_____
DAY 6	_____	_____	_____
DAY 7	_____	_____	_____
TOTALS	_____	_____	_____

DAY 1

FOOD TRACKING

DESCRIPTION   **CALORIE/**
                           FAT/CARB

_____   _____

_____   _____

_____   _____

_____   _____

_____   _____

_____   _____

_____   _____

_____   _____

_____   _____

_____   _____

_____   _____

_____   _____

_____   _____

_____   _____

_____   _____

TOTALS   _____

GLASSES OF WATER CHECK-LIST

☐   ☐   ☐   ☐

☐   ☐   ☐   ☐

DAILY EXERCISES (SEE EXERCISE LIST)

DESCRIPTION   **TIME**

_____   ____

_____   ____

_____   ____

_____   ____

_____   ____

_____   ____

NOTES

_____

_____

_____

_____

_____

_____

_____

DAY 2

FOOD TRACKING

DESCRIPTION	CALORIE/ FAT/CARB
_____	_____
_____	_____
_____	_____
_____	_____
_____	_____
_____	_____
_____	_____
_____	_____
_____	_____
_____	_____
_____	_____
_____	_____
_____	_____
_____	_____
_____	_____
_____	_____

GLASSES OF WATER CHECK-LIST

☐ ☐ ☐ ☐

☐ ☐ ☐ ☐

DAILY EXERCISES (SEE EXERCISE LIST)

DESCRIPTION	TIME
_____	_____
_____	_____
_____	_____
_____	_____
_____	_____
_____	_____

NOTES

_____

_____

_____

_____

_____

_____

_____

TOTALS _____

DAY 3

FOOD TRACKING

DESCRIPTION	CALORIE/ FAT/CARB
_____	_____
_____	_____
_____	_____
_____	_____
_____	_____
_____	_____
_____	_____
_____	_____
_____	_____
_____	_____
_____	_____
_____	_____
_____	_____
_____	_____
_____	_____
_____	_____
_____	_____

TOTALS _____

GLASSES OF WATER CHECK-LIST

☐ ☐ ☐ ☐

☐ ☐ ☐ ☐

DAILY EXERCISES (SEE EXERCISE LIST)

DESCRIPTION	TIME
_____	____
_____	____
_____	____
_____	____
_____	____
_____	____

NOTES

_____

_____

_____

_____

_____

_____

_____

DAY 4

FOOD TRACKING

DESCRIPTION   **CALORIE/ FAT/CARB**

_____   _____

_____   _____

_____   _____

_____   _____

_____   _____

_____   _____

_____   _____

_____   _____

_____   _____

_____   _____

_____   _____

_____   _____

_____   _____

_____   _____

_____   _____

TOTALS   _____

GLASSES OF WATER CHECK-LIST

☐ ☐ ☐ ☐

☐ ☐ ☐ ☐

DAILY EXERCISES (SEE EXERCISE LIST)

DESCRIPTION   **TIME**

_____   _____

_____   _____

_____   _____

_____   _____

_____   _____

_____   _____

NOTES

_____

_____

_____

_____

_____

_____

_____

DAY 5

FOOD TRACKING

DESCRIPTION	CALORIE/ FAT/CARB
_____	_____
_____	_____
_____	_____
_____	_____
_____	_____
_____	_____
_____	_____
_____	_____
_____	_____
_____	_____
_____	_____
_____	_____
_____	_____
_____	_____
_____	_____
_____	_____

TOTALS _____

GLASSES OF WATER CHECK-LIST

☐ ☐ ☐ ☐

☐ ☐ ☐ ☐

DAILY EXERCISES (SEE EXERCISE LIST)

DESCRIPTION	TIME
_____	_____
_____	_____
_____	_____
_____	_____
_____	_____
_____	_____

NOTES

_____

_____

_____

_____

_____

_____

_____

DAY 6

FOOD TRACKING

DESCRIPTION   **CALORIE/ FAT/CARB**

_____   _____

_____   _____

_____   _____

_____   _____

_____   _____

_____   _____

_____   _____

_____   _____

_____   _____

_____   _____

_____   _____

_____   _____

_____   _____

_____   _____

_____   _____

_____   _____

TOTALS   _____

GLASSES OF WATER CHECK-LIST

☐   ☐   ☐   ☐

☐   ☐   ☐   ☐

DAILY EXERCISES (SEE EXERCISE LIST)

DESCRIPTION   **TIME**

_____   _____

_____   _____

_____   _____

_____   _____

_____   _____

_____   _____

NOTES

_____

_____

_____

_____

_____

_____

_____

DAY 7

FOOD TRACKING

DESCRIPTION	CALORIE/ FAT/CARB
_____	_____
_____	_____
_____	_____
_____	_____
_____	_____
_____	_____
_____	_____
_____	_____
_____	_____
_____	_____
_____	_____
_____	_____
_____	_____
_____	_____
_____	_____
_____	_____
_____	_____

TOTALS _____

GLASSES OF WATER CHECK-LIST

☐ ☐ ☐ ☐

☐ ☐ ☐ ☐

DAILY EXERCISES (SEE EXERCISE LIST)

DESCRIPTION	TIME
_____	_____
_____	_____
_____	_____
_____	_____
_____	_____
_____	_____

NOTES

_____

_____

_____

_____

_____

_____

_____

WEEKLY TOTALS

	CALORIES FAT OR CARBS	WATER	EXERCISE TIME
DAY 1	_____	_____	_____
DAY 2	_____	_____	_____
DAY 3	_____	_____	_____
DAY 4	_____	_____	_____
DAY 5	_____	_____	_____
DAY 6	_____	_____	_____
DAY 7	_____	_____	_____
TOTALS	_____	_____	_____

DAY 1

FOOD TRACKING

DESCRIPTION   **CALORIE/**
                                   FAT/CARB

_____   _____

_____   _____

_____   _____

_____   _____

_____   _____

_____   _____

_____   _____

_____   _____

_____   _____

_____   _____

_____   _____

_____   _____

_____   _____

_____   _____

TOTALS   _____

GLASSES OF WATER CHECK-LIST

☐   ☐   ☐   ☐

☐   ☐   ☐   ☐

DAILY EXERCISES (SEE EXERCISE LIST)

DESCRIPTION   **TIME**

_____   _____

_____   _____

_____   _____

_____   _____

_____   _____

_____   _____

NOTES

_____

_____

_____

_____

_____

_____

_____

DAY 2

FOOD TRACKING

DESCRIPTION	CALORIE/ FAT/CARB
_____	_____
_____	_____
_____	_____
_____	_____
_____	_____
_____	_____
_____	_____
_____	_____
_____	_____
_____	_____
_____	_____
_____	_____
_____	_____
_____	_____
_____	_____
_____	_____
_____	_____

TOTALS _____

GLASSES OF WATER CHECK-LIST

☐ ☐ ☐ ☐

☐ ☐ ☐ ☐

DAILY EXERCISES (SEE EXERCISE LIST)

DESCRIPTION	TIME
_____	_____
_____	_____
_____	_____
_____	_____
_____	_____
_____	_____

NOTES

_____

_____

_____

_____

_____

_____

_____

DAY 3

FOOD TRACKING

DESCRIPTION	CALORIE/ FAT/CARB
_____	_____
_____	_____
_____	_____
_____	_____
_____	_____
_____	_____
_____	_____
_____	_____
_____	_____
_____	_____
_____	_____
_____	_____
_____	_____
_____	_____
_____	_____

GLASSES OF WATER CHECK-LIST

☐ ☐ ☐ ☐

☐ ☐ ☐ ☐

DAILY EXERCISES (SEE EXERCISE LIST)

DESCRIPTION	TIME
_____	_____
_____	_____
_____	_____
_____	_____
_____	_____
_____	_____

NOTES

_____

_____

_____

_____

_____

_____

_____

_____

TOTALS _____

DAY 4

FOOD TRACKING

DESCRIPTION	CALORIE/ FAT/CARB
_____	_____
_____	_____
_____	_____
_____	_____
_____	_____
_____	_____
_____	_____
_____	_____
_____	_____
_____	_____
_____	_____
_____	_____
_____	_____
_____	_____
_____	_____
_____	_____

TOTALS _____

GLASSES OF WATER CHECK-LIST

☐ ☐ ☐ ☐
☐ ☐ ☐ ☐

DAILY EXERCISES (SEE EXERCISE LIST)

DESCRIPTION	TIME
_____	____
_____	____
_____	____
_____	____
_____	____
_____	____

NOTES

_____
_____
_____
_____
_____
_____
_____

DAY 5

FOOD TRACKING

DESCRIPTION   **CALORIE/**
                         FAT/CARB

_____ _____

_____ _____

_____ _____

_____ _____

_____ _____

_____ _____

_____ _____

_____ _____

_____ _____

_____ _____

_____ _____

_____ _____

_____ _____

_____ _____

_____ _____

_____ _____

TOTALS   _____

GLASSES OF WATER CHECK-LIST

☐   ☐   ☐   ☐

☐   ☐   ☐   ☐

DAILY EXERCISES (SEE EXERCISE LIST)

DESCRIPTION   **TIME**

_____   _____

_____   _____

_____   _____

_____   _____

_____   _____

_____   _____

NOTES

_____

_____

_____

_____

_____

_____

_____

DAY 6

FOOD TRACKING

DESCRIPTION	CALORIE/ FAT/CARB
_____	_____
_____	_____
_____	_____
_____	_____
_____	_____
_____	_____
_____	_____
_____	_____
_____	_____
_____	_____
_____	_____
_____	_____
_____	_____
_____	_____
_____	_____

TOTALS _____

GLASSES OF WATER CHECK-LIST

☐ ☐ ☐ ☐

☐ ☐ ☐ ☐

DAILY EXERCISES (SEE EXERCISE LIST)

DESCRIPTION	TIME
_____	_____
_____	_____
_____	_____
_____	_____
_____	_____
_____	_____

NOTES

_____

_____

_____

_____

_____

_____

_____

DAY 7

FOOD TRACKING

DESCRIPTION	CALORIE/ FAT/CARB
_____	_____
_____	_____
_____	_____
_____	_____
_____	_____
_____	_____
_____	_____
_____	_____
_____	_____
_____	_____
_____	_____
_____	_____
_____	_____
_____	_____
_____	_____
_____	_____
_____	_____
_____	_____

TOTALS _____

GLASSES OF WATER CHECK-LIST

☐ ☐ ☐ ☐

☐ ☐ ☐ ☐

DAILY EXERCISES (SEE EXERCISE LIST)

DESCRIPTION	TIME
_____	_____
_____	_____
_____	_____
_____	_____
_____	_____
_____	_____

NOTES

_____

_____

_____

_____

_____

_____

_____

WEEKLY TOTALS

	CALORIES FAT OR CARBS	WATER	EXERCISE TIME
DAY 1	_____	_____	_____
DAY 2	_____	_____	_____
DAY 3	_____	_____	_____
DAY 4	_____	_____	_____
DAY 5	_____	_____	_____
DAY 6	_____	_____	_____
DAY 7	_____	_____	_____
TOTALS	_____	_____	_____

DAY 1

FOOD TRACKING

DESCRIPTION	CALORIE/ FAT/CARB
_____	_____
_____	_____
_____	_____
_____	_____
_____	_____
_____	_____
_____	_____
_____	_____
_____	_____
_____	_____
_____	_____
_____	_____
_____	_____
_____	_____

TOTALS _____

GLASSES OF WATER CHECK-LIST

☐ ☐ ☐ ☐

☐ ☐ ☐ ☐

DAILY EXERCISES (SEE EXERCISE LIST)

DESCRIPTION	TIME
_____	_____
_____	_____
_____	_____
_____	_____
_____	_____
_____	_____

NOTES

_____

_____

_____

_____

_____

_____

_____

DAY 2

FOOD TRACKING

DESCRIPTION	CALORIE/ FAT/CARB
_____	_____
_____	_____
_____	_____
_____	_____
_____	_____
_____	_____
_____	_____
_____	_____
_____	_____
_____	_____
_____	_____
_____	_____
_____	_____
_____	_____

TOTALS _____

GLASSES OF WATER CHECK-LIST

☐ ☐ ☐ ☐

☐ ☐ ☐ ☐

DAILY EXERCISES (SEE EXERCISE LIST)

DESCRIPTION	TIME
_____	____
_____	____
_____	____
_____	____
_____	____

NOTES

_____

_____

_____

_____

_____

_____

_____

DAY 3

FOOD TRACKING

DESCRIPTION	CALORIE/ FAT/CARB
_____	____
_____	____
_____	____
_____	____
_____	____
_____	____
_____	____
_____	____
_____	____
_____	____
_____	____
_____	____
_____	____
_____	____
_____	____
_____	____

TOTALS _____

GLASSES OF WATER CHECK-LIST

☐ ☐ ☐ ☐

☐ ☐ ☐ ☐

DAILY EXERCISES (SEE EXERCISE LIST)

DESCRIPTION	TIME
_____	____
_____	____
_____	____
_____	____
_____	____
_____	____

NOTES

_____

_____

_____

_____

_____

_____

_____

DAY 4

FOOD TRACKING

DESCRIPTION	CALORIE/ FAT/CARB
_____	_____
_____	_____
_____	_____
_____	_____
_____	_____
_____	_____
_____	_____
_____	_____
_____	_____
_____	_____
_____	_____
_____	_____
_____	_____
_____	_____
_____	_____
_____	_____
_____	_____

TOTALS _____

GLASSES OF WATER CHECK-LIST

☐ ☐ ☐ ☐

☐ ☐ ☐ ☐

DAILY EXERCISES (SEE EXERCISE LIST)

DESCRIPTION	TIME
_____	_____
_____	_____
_____	_____
_____	_____
_____	_____
_____	_____

NOTES

_____

_____

_____

_____

_____

_____

_____

DAY 5

FOOD TRACKING

DESCRIPTION   **CALORIE/**
                               FAT/CARB

_____ _____

_____ _____

_____ _____

_____ _____

_____ _____

_____ _____

_____ _____

_____ _____

_____ _____

_____ _____

_____ _____

_____ _____

_____ _____

_____ _____

_____ _____

_____ _____

_____ _____

_____ _____

TOTALS _____

GLASSES OF WATER CHECK-LIST

☐   ☐   ☐   ☐

☐   ☐   ☐   ☐

DAILY EXERCISES (SEE EXERCISE LIST)

DESCRIPTION   **TIME**

_____ ____

_____ ____

_____ ____

_____ ____

_____ ____

_____ ____

NOTES

_____

_____

_____

_____

_____

_____

DAY 6

FOOD TRACKING

DESCRIPTION   **CALORIE/ FAT/CARB**

_____   _____

_____   _____

_____   _____

_____   _____

_____   _____

_____   _____

_____   _____

_____   _____

_____   _____

_____   _____

_____   _____

_____   _____

_____   _____

_____   _____

_____   _____

_____   _____

TOTALS   _____

GLASSES OF WATER CHECK-LIST

☐   ☐   ☐   ☐

☐   ☐   ☐   ☐

DAILY EXERCISES (SEE EXERCISE LIST)

DESCRIPTION   **TIME**

_____   ____

_____   ____

_____   ____

_____   ____

_____   ____

_____   ____

NOTES

_____

_____

_____

_____

_____

_____

_____

_____

DAY 7

FOOD TRACKING

DESCRIPTION

CALORIE/ FAT/CARB

_____ _____

_____ _____

_____ _____

_____ _____

_____ _____

_____ _____

_____ _____

_____ _____

_____ _____

_____ _____

_____ _____

_____ _____

_____ _____

_____ _____

_____ _____

_____ _____

_____ _____

TOTALS _____

GLASSES OF WATER CHECK-LIST

☐ ☐ ☐ ☐

☐ ☐ ☐ ☐

DAILY EXERCISES (SEE EXERCISE LIST)

DESCRIPTION   **TIME**

_____ ____

_____ ____

_____ ____

_____ ____

_____ ____

_____ ____

NOTES

_____

_____

_____

_____

_____

_____

_____

WEEKLY TOTALS

	CALORIES FAT OR CARBS	WATER	EXERCISE TIME
DAY 1	_____	_____	_____
DAY 2	_____	_____	_____
DAY 3	_____	_____	_____
DAY 4	_____	_____	_____
DAY 5	_____	_____	_____
DAY 6	_____	_____	_____
DAY 7	_____	_____	_____
TOTALS	_____	_____	_____

EXERCISE LIST

VARY YOUR EXERCISING SO YOU'LL STICK TO IT

AEROBICS

ARCHERY

BACKPACKING

BADMINTON

BASKETBALL

BICYCLING

BOWLING

BOXING

CANOEING

CLEANING HOUSE

CRICKET

CROQUET

CURLING

DANCING

DARTS

DIVING

FISHING

FOOTBALL

GARDENING

GOLF

HICKING

HOCKEY

HORSEBACK RIDING

JAI ALAI

JOGGING

KAYAKING

LACROSSE

MOWING LAWN

POLO

POWER WALKING

RAKING LEAVES

ROCK CLIMBING

ROWING

RUNNING

SAILING

SHOVELING SNOW

SKATEBOARDING

SKATING

SKIING

SCUBA DIVING

SLEDDING

SNOW SHOEING

SOCCER

SOFTBALL

SQUASH

STRETCHING

SWIMMING

TABLE TENNIS

TENNIS

VOLLEYBALL

WALKING

WEIGHT LIFTING

WHITEWATER RAFTING

YOGA

CHART BY FOOD CATEGORY

CHART BY FOOD CATEGORY

		Fat Grams	Food Energy Calories	Carbohydrate Grams
BEVERAGES	Apple juice, canned 1 cup	0	115	29
BEVERAGES	Beer, light 12 fl oz	0	95	5
BEVERAGES	Beer, regular 12 fl oz	0	150	13
BEVERAGES	Chocolate milk, lowfat 1% 1 cup	3	160	26
BEVERAGES	Chocolate milk, lowfat 2% 1 cup	5	180	26
BEVERAGES	Chocolate milk, regular 1 cup	8	210	26
BEVERAGES	Club soda 12 fl oz	0	0	0
BEVERAGES	Coffee, brewed 6 fl oz	0	0	0
BEVERAGES	Coffee, instant, prepared 6 fl oz	0	0	1
BEVERAGES	Cola, diet, aspartame only 12 fl oz	0	0	0
BEVERAGES	Cola, diet, asprtame + sacchrn12 fl oz	0	0	0
BEVERAGES	Cola, diet, saccharin only 12 fl oz	0	0	0
BEVERAGES	Cola, regular 12 fl oz	0	160	41
BEVERAGES	Cranberry juice cocktal w/vitc1 cup	0	145	38
BEVERAGES	Eggnog 1 cup	19	340	34
BEVERAGES	Evaporated milk, skim, canned 1 cup	1	200	29
BEVERAGES	Evaporated milk, whole, canned1 cup	19	340	25
BEVERAGES	Fruit punch drink, canned 6 fl oz	0	85	22
BEVERAGES	Gin,rum,vodka,whisky 80-proof 1.5 f oz	0	95	0
BEVERAGES	Gin,rum,vodka,whisky 86-proof 1.5 f oz	0	105	0
BEVERAGES	Gin,rum,vodka,whisky 90-proof 1.5 f oz	0	110	0
BEVERAGES	Ginger ale 12 fl oz	0	125	32
BEVERAGES	Grape drink, canned 6 fl oz	0	100	26
BEVERAGES	Grape juice, canned 1 cup	0	155	38
BEVERAGES	Grape soda 12 fl oz	0	180	46
BEVERAGES	Grapefrt jce,frzn,cncn,unswten6 fl oz	1	300	72
BEVERAGES	Grapefrt jce,frzn,dltd,unswten1 cup	0	100	24
BEVERAGES	Grapefruit juice, canned,swtnd1 cup	0	115	28
BEVERAGES	Grapefruit juice, canned,unswt1 cup	0	95	22
BEVERAGES	Grapefruit juice, raw 1 cup	0	95	23
BEVERAGES	Grapefruit, canned, syrup pack1 cup	0	150	39
BEVERAGES	Grapefruit, raw, pink 1/2 frut	0	40	10
BEVERAGES	Grapefruit, raw, white 1/2 frut	0	40	10
BEVERAGES	Grapejce,frzn,concen,swtnd,w/c6 fl oz	1	385	96
BEVERAGES	Grapejce,frzn,dilutd,swtnd,w/c1 cup	0	125	32
BEVERAGES	Half and half, cream 1 cup	28	315	10
BEVERAGES	Half and half, cream 1 tbsp	2	20	1

CHART BY FOOD CATEGORY

		Fat Grams	Food Energy Calories	Carbohydrate Grams
BEVERAGES	Lemon juice,frzn,single-strngh6 fl oz	1	55	16
BEVERAGES	Lemonade,concen,frzen,diluted 6 fl oz	0	80	21
BEVERAGES	Lemonade,concentrate,frz,undil6 fl oz	0	425	112
BEVERAGES	Lemon-lime soda 12 fl oz	0	155	39
BEVERAGES	Limeade,concen,frozen,diluted 6 fl oz	0	75	20
BEVERAGES	Limeade,concentrate,frzn,undil6 fl oz	0	410	108
BEVERAGES	Orange + grapefruit juce,cannd1 cup	0	105	25
BEVERAGES	Orange juice, canned 1 cup	0	105	25
BEVERAGES	Orange juice, chilled 1 cup	1	110	25
BEVERAGES	Orange juice, raw 1 cup	0	110	26
BEVERAGES	Orange juice,frozen concentrte6 fl oz	0	340	81
BEVERAGES	Orange juice,frzn,cncn,diluted1 cup	0	110	27
BEVERAGES	Pepper-type soda 12 fl oz	0	160	41
BEVERAGES	Pineapple juice, canned,unswtn1 cup	0	140	34
BEVERAGES	Pineapple-grapefruit juicedrnk6 fl oz	0	90	23
BEVERAGES	Root beer 12 fl oz	0	165	42
BEVERAGES	Tea, brewed 8 fl oz	0	0	0
BEVERAGES	Tea, instant,preprd,unsweetend8 fl oz	0	0	1
BEVERAGES	Tea,instant,prepard,sweetened 8 fl oz	0	85	22
BEVERAGES	Tomato juice, canned w/o salt 1 cup	0	40	10
BEVERAGES	Tomato juice, canned with salt1 cup	0	40	10
BEVERAGES	Vegetable juice cocktail, cnnd1 cup	0	45	11
BEVERAGES	Wine, dessert 3.5 f oz	0	140	8
BEVERAGES	Wine, table, red 3.5 f oz	0	75	3
BEVERAGES	Wine, table, white 3.5 f oz	0	80	3
BREADS	Bagels, egg 1 bagel	2	200	38
BREADS	Bagels, plain 1 bagel	2	200	38
BREADS	Baking powder,sas,capo4+caso4 1 tsp	0	5	1
BREADS	Baking pwdr biscuits,from mix 1 biscut	3	95	14
BREADS	Baking pwdr biscuits,homerecpe1 biscut	5	100	13
BREADS	Baking pwdr biscuits,refrgdogh1 biscut	2	65	10
BREADS	Boston brown bread,w/whtecrnm 1 slice	1	95	21
BREADS	Boston brown bread,w/yllwcrnml1 slice	1	95	21
BREADS	Bran muffins, from commerl mix1 muffin	4	140	24
BREADS	Bran muffins, home recipe 1 muffin	6	125	19
BREADS	Bread stuffing,from mx,drytype1 cup	31	500	50
BREADS	Bread stuffing,from mx,moist 1 cup	26	420	40
BREADS	Breadcrumbs, dry, grated 1 cup	5	390	73
BREADS	Cheese crackers, plain 10 crack	3	50	6
BREADS	Cheese crackers, sandwch,peant1 sandwh	2	40	5
BREADS	Coffeecake, crumb, from mix 1 cake	41	1385	225

CHART BY FOOD CATEGORY

		Fat Grams	Food Energy Calories	Carbohydrate Grams
BREADS	Coffeecake, crumb, from mix 1 piece	7	230	38
BREADS	Corn chips 1 oz	9	155	16
BREADS	Corn grits, cooked, instant 1 pkt	0	80	18
BREADS	Corn grits,ckd,reg,whte,nosalt1 cup	0	145	31
BREADS	Corn grits,ckd,reg,whte,w/salt1 cup	0	145	31
BREADS	Corn grits,ckd,reg,yllw,nosalt1 cup	0	145	31
BREADS	Corn grits,ckd,reg,yllw,w/salt1 cup	0	145	31
BREADS	Corn muffins, from commerl mix1 muffin	6	145	22
BREADS	Cornmeal,bolted,dry form 1 cup	4	440	91
BREADS	Cornmeal,degermed,enrched,cook1 cup	0	120	26
BREADS	Cornmeal,degermed,enriched,dry1 cup	2	500	108
BREADS	Cornmeal,whole-grnd,unbolt,dry1 cup	5	435	90
BREADS	Cracked-wheat bread 1 loaf	16	1190	227
BREADS	Cracked-wheat bread 1 slice	1	65	12
BREADS	Cracked-wheat bread, toasted 1 slice	1	65	12
BREADS	Croissants 1 crosst	12	235	27
BREADS	Danish pastry, fruit 1 pastry	13	235	28
BREADS	Danish pastry, plain, no nuts 1 oz	6	110	13
BREADS	Danish pastry, plain, no nuts 1 pastry	12	220	26
BREADS	Danish pastry, plain, no nuts 1 ring	71	1305	152
BREADS	Enchilada 1 enchld	16	235	24
BREADS	Eng muffin, egg, cheese, bacon1 sandwh	18	360	31
BREADS	English muffins, plain 1 muffin	1	140	27
BREADS	English muffins, plain, toastd1 muffin	1	140	27
BREADS	French bread 1 slice	1	100	18
BREADS	French or vienna bread 1 loaf	18	1270	230
BREADS	French toast, home recipe 1 slice	7	155	17
BREADS	Italian bread 1 loaf	4	1255	256
BREADS	Italian bread 1 slice	0	85	17
BREADS	Lucky charms cereal 1 oz	1	110	23
BREADS	Melba toast, plain 1 piece	0	20	4
BREADS	Mixed grain bread 1 loaf	17	1165	212
BREADS	Mixed grain bread 1 slice	1	65	12
BREADS	Mixed grain bread, toasted 1 slice	1	65	12
BREADS	Oatmeal bread 1 loaf	20	1145	212
BREADS	Oatmeal bread 1 slice	1	65	12
BREADS	Oatmeal bread, toasted 1 slice	1	65	12
BREADS	Oatmeal w/ raisins cookies 4 cookie	10	245	36
BREADS	Oatmeal,ckd,instnt,flvrd,fortf1 pkt	2	160	31
BREADS	Oatmeal,ckd,instnt,plain,fortf1 pkt	2	105	18
BREADS	Oatmeal,ckd,rg,qck,inst,w/osal1 cup	2	145	25

CHART BY FOOD CATEGORY

		Fat Grams	Food Energy Calories	Carbohydrate Grams
BREADS	Oatmeal,ckd,rg,qck,inst,w/salt1 cup	2	145	25
BREADS	Pancakes, buckwheat, from mix 1 pancak	2	55	6
BREADS	Pancakes, plain, from mix 1 pancak	2	60	8
BREADS	Pancakes, plain, home recipe 1 pancak	2	60	9
BREADS	Piecrust, from mix 2 crust	93	1485	141
BREADS	Piecrust,from home recipe 1 shell	60	900	79
BREADS	Pita bread 1 pita	1	165	33
BREADS	Pizza, cheese 1 slice	9	290	39
BREADS	Potato chips 10 chips	7	105	10
BREADS	Pretzels, stick 10 pretz	0	10	2
BREADS	Pretzels, twisted, dutch 1 pretz	1	65	13
BREADS	Pretzels, twisted, thin 10 pretz	2	240	48
BREADS	Pumpernickel bread 1 loaf	16	1160	218
BREADS	Pumpernickel bread 1 slice	1	80	16
BREADS	Pumpernickel bread, toasted 1 slice	1	80	16
BREADS	Raisin bread 1 loaf	18	1260	239
BREADS	Raisin bread 1 slice	1	65	13
BREADS	Raisin bread, toasted 1 slice	1	65	13
BREADS	Rice krispies cereal 1 oz	0	110	25
BREADS	Rolls, dinner, commercial 1 roll	2	85	14
BREADS	Rolls, dinner, home recipe 1 roll	3	120	20
BREADS	Rolls, frankfurter + hamburger1 roll	2	115	20
BREADS	Rolls, hard 1 roll	2	155	30
BREADS	Rolls, hoagie or submarine 1 roll	8	400	72
BREADS	Rye bread, light 1 loaf	17	1190	218
BREADS	Rye bread, light 1 slice	1	65	12
BREADS	Rye bread, light, toasted 1 slice	1	65	12
BREADS	Rye wafers, whole-grain 2 wafers	1	55	10
BREADS	Saltines 4 crackr	1	50	9
BREADS	Sandwich spread, pork, beef 1 tbsp	3	35	2
BREADS	Self-rising flour, unsifted 1 cup	1	440	93
BREADS	Snack type crackers 1 crackr	1	15	2
BREADS	Taco 1 taco	11	195	15
BREADS	Toaster pastries 1 pastry	6	210	38
BREADS	Tortillas, corn 1 tortla	1	65	13
BREADS	Vienna bread 1 slice	1	70	13
BREADS	Waffles, from home recipe 1 waffle	13	245	26
BREADS	Waffles, from mix 1 waffle	8	205	27
BREADS	Wheat bread 1 loaf	19	1160	213
BREADS	Wheat bread 1 slice	1	65	12
BREADS	Wheat bread, toasted 1 slice	1	65	12

CHART BY FOOD CATEGORY

		Fat Grams	Food Energy Calories	Carbohydrate Grams
BREADS	Wheat flour, all-purpose,siftd1 cup	1	420	88
BREADS	Wheat flour, all-purpose,unsif1 cup	1	455	95
BREADS	Wheat, thin crackers 4 crackr	1	35	5
BREADS	White bread 1 loaf	18	1210	222
BREADS	White bread crumbs, soft 1 cup	2	120	22
BREADS	White bread cubes 1 cup	1	80	15
BREADS	White bread, slice 18 per loaf1 slice	1	65	12
BREADS	White bread, slice 22 per loaf1 slice	1	55	10
BREADS	White bread, toasted 18 per 1 slice	1	65	12
BREADS	White bread, toasted 22 per 1 slice	1	55	10
CEREAL	100% natural cereal 1 oz	6	135	18
CEREAL	All-bran cereal 1 oz	1	70	21
CEREAL	Bran flakes, kellogg's 1 oz	1	90	22
CEREAL	Bran flakes, post 1 oz	0	90	22
CEREAL	Cap'n crunch cereal 1 oz	3	120	23
CEREAL	Cheerios cereal 1 oz	2	110	20
CEREAL	Corn flakes, kellogg's 1 oz	0	110	24
CEREAL	Corn flakes, toasties 1 oz	0	110	24
CEREAL	Froot loops cereal 1 oz	1	110	25
CEREAL	Golden grahams cereal 1 oz	1	110	24
CEREAL	Grape-nuts cereal 1 oz	0	100	23
CEREAL	Honey nut cheerios cereal 1 oz	1	105	23
CEREAL	Nature valley granola cereal 1 oz	5	125	19
CEREAL	Product 19 cereal 1 oz	0	110	24
CEREAL	Raisin bran, kellogg's 1 oz	1	90	21
CEREAL	Raisin bran, post 1 oz	1	85	21
CEREAL	Shredded wheat cereal 1 oz	1	100	23
CEREAL	Special k cereal 1 oz	0	110	21
CEREAL	Sugar frosted flakes, kellogg 1 oz	0	110	26
CEREAL	Sugar smacks cereal 1 oz	1	105	25
CEREAL	Super sugar crisp cereal 1 oz	0	105	26
CEREAL	Total cereal 1 oz	1	100	22
CEREAL	Trix cereal 1 oz	0	110	25
CEREAL	Wheaties cereal 1 oz	0	100	23
DAIRY	Blue cheese 1 oz	8	100	1
DAIRY	Butter, salted 1 pat	4	35	0
DAIRY	Butter, salted 1 tbsp	11	100	0
DAIRY	Butter, salted 1/2 cup	92	810	0
DAIRY	Butter, unsalted 1 pat	4	35	0
DAIRY	Butter, unsalted 1 tbsp	11	100	0
DAIRY	Butter, unsalted 1/2 cup	92	810	0

CHART BY FOOD CATEGORY

			Fat Grams	Food Energy Calories	Carbohydrate Grams
DAIRY	Buttermilk, dried	1 cup	7	465	59
DAIRY	Buttermilk, fluid	1 cup	2	100	12
DAIRY	Camembert cheese	1 wedge	9	115	0
DAIRY	Cheddar cheese	1 cu in	6	70	0
DAIRY	Cheddar cheese	1 oz	9	115	0
DAIRY	Chedddar cheese, shredded	1 cup	37	455	1
DAIRY	Cheese sauce w/ milk, frm mix 1 cup		17	305	23
DAIRY	Cottage cheese,cremd,lrge curd1 cup		10	235	6
DAIRY	Cottage cheese,cremd,smll curd1 cup		9	215	6
DAIRY	Cottage cheese,cremd,w/fruit	1 cup	8	280	30
DAIRY	Cottage cheese,lowfat 2%	1 cup	4	205	8
DAIRY	Cottage cheese,uncreamed	1 cup	1	125	3
DAIRY	Cream cheese	1 oz	10	100	1
DAIRY	Cream of wheat,ckd,mix n eat	1 pkt	0	100	21
DAIRY	Crm wheat,ckd, quick, no salt 1 cup		0	140	29
DAIRY	Crm wheat,ckd,quick, w/ salt 1 cup		0	140	29
DAIRY	Crm wheat,ckd,reg,inst,no salt1 cup		0	140	29
DAIRY	Crm wheat,ckd,reg,inst,w/salt 1 cup		0	140	29
DAIRY	Eggs, cooked, fried	1 egg	7	90	1
DAIRY	Eggs, cooked, hard-cooked	1 egg	5	75	1
DAIRY	Eggs, cooked, poached	1 egg	5	75	1
DAIRY	Eggs, cooked, scrambled/omelet1 egg		7	100	1
DAIRY	Eggs, raw, white	1 white	0	15	0
DAIRY	Eggs, raw, whole	1 egg	5	75	1
DAIRY	Eggs, raw, yolk	1 yolk	5	60	0
DAIRY	Feta cheese	1 oz	6	75	1
DAIRY	Ice cream, vanlla, regulr 11% 1 cup		14	270	32
DAIRY	Ice cream, vanlla, regulr 11% 1/2 galn		115	2155	254
DAIRY	Ice cream, vanlla, regulr 11% 3 fl oz		5	100	12
DAIRY	Ice cream, vanlla, rich 16% ft1 cup		24	350	32
DAIRY	Ice cream, vanlla, rich 16% ft1/2 gal		190	2805	256
DAIRY	Ice cream, vanlla, soft serve 1 cup		23	375	38
DAIRY	Ice milk, vanilla, 4% fat	1 cup	6	185	29
DAIRY	Ice milk, vanilla, 4% fat	1/2 gal	45	1470	232
DAIRY	Ice milk, vanilla,softserv 3% 1 cup		5	225	38
DAIRY	Imitation creamers, liquid frz1 tbsp		1	20	2
DAIRY	Imitation creamers, powdered	1 tsp	1	10	1
DAIRY	Imitation whipped topping,frzn1 cup		19	240	17
DAIRY	Imitation whipped topping,frzn1 tbsp		1	15	1
DAIRY	Imitatn sour dressing	1 cup	39	415	11
DAIRY	Imitatn sour dressing	1 tbsp	2	20	1

CHART BY FOOD CATEGORY

		Fat Grams	Food Energy Calories	Carbohydrate Grams
DAIRY	Imitatn whipd toping,pressrzd 1 cup	16	185	11
DAIRY	Imitatn whipd toping,pressrzd 1 tbsp	1	10	1
DAIRY	Imitatn whipd toping,pwdrd,prp1 cup	10	150	13
DAIRY	Imitatn whipd toping,pwdrd,prp1 tbsp	0	10	1
DAIRY	Lard 1 cup	205	1850	0
DAIRY	Lard 1 tbsp	13	115	0
DAIRY	Light, coffee or table cream 1 cup	46	470	9
DAIRY	Light, coffee or table cream 1 tbsp	3	30	1
DAIRY	Malted milk, chocolate, powder3/4 oz	1	85	18
DAIRY	Malted milk,chocolate, pwdrppd1 servng	9	235	29
DAIRY	Malted milk,natural, powder 3/4 oz	2	85	15
DAIRY	Malted milk,natural, pwdr pprd1 servng	10	235	27
DAIRY	Margarine, imitation 40% fat 1 tbsp	5	50	0
DAIRY	Margarine, imitation 40% fat 8 oz	88	785	1
DAIRY	Margarine, regulr,hard,80% fat1 pat	4	35	0
DAIRY	Margarine, regulr,hard,80% fat1 tbsp	11	100	0
DAIRY	Margarine, regulr,hard,80% fat1/2 cup	91	810	1
DAIRY	Margarine, regulr,soft,80% fat1 tbsp	11	100	0
DAIRY	Margarine, regulr,soft,80% fat8 oz	183	1625	1
DAIRY	Margarine, spread,hard,60% fat1 pat	3	25	0
DAIRY	Margarine, spread,hard,60% fat1 tbsp	9	75	0
DAIRY	Margarine, spread,hard,60% fat1/2 cup	69	610	0
DAIRY	Margarine, spread,soft,60% fat1 tbsp	9	75	0
DAIRY	Margarine, spread,soft,60% fat8 oz	138	1225	0
DAIRY	Milk, lofat, 1%, added solids 1 cup	2	105	12
DAIRY	Milk, lofat, 1%, no addedsolid1 cup	3	100	12
DAIRY	Milk, lofat, 2%, added solids 1 cup	5	125	12
DAIRY	Milk, lofat, 2%, no addedsolid1 cup	5	120	12
DAIRY	Milk, skim, added milk solids 1 cup	1	90	12
DAIRY	Milk, skim, no added milksolid1 cup	0	85	12
DAIRY	Milk, whole, 3.3% fat 1 cup	8	150	11
DAIRY	Mozzarella cheese, whole milk 1 oz	6	80	1
DAIRY	Mozzarella chese,skim, lomoist1 oz	5	80	1
DAIRY	Muenster cheese 1 oz	9	105	0
DAIRY	Nonfat dry milk, instantized 1 cup	0	245	35
DAIRY	Nonfat dry milk, instantized 1 envlpe	1	325	47
DAIRY	Parmesan cheese, grated 1 cup	30	455	4
DAIRY	Parmesan cheese, grated 1 oz	9	130	1
DAIRY	Parmesan cheese, grated 1 tbsp	2	25	0
DAIRY	Pasterzd proces cheese, swiss 1 oz	7	95	1
DAIRY	Pasterzd proces cheese,americn1 oz	9	105	0

CHART BY FOOD CATEGORY

		Fat Grams	Food Energy Calories	Carbohydrate Grams
DAIRY	Pasterzd proces chese food,amr1 oz	7	95	2
DAIRY	Pasterzd proces chese spred,am1 oz	6	80	2
DAIRY	Provolone cheese 1 oz	8	100	1
DAIRY	Pudding, choc, cooked from mix1/2 cup	4	150	25
DAIRY	Pudding, choc, instant, fr mix1/2 cup	4	155	27
DAIRY	Pudding, chocolate,canned 5 oz	11	205	30
DAIRY	Pudding, rice, from mix 1/2 cup	4	155	27
DAIRY	Pudding, tapioca, canned 5 oz	5	160	28
DAIRY	Pudding, tapioca, from mix 1/2 cup	4	145	25
DAIRY	Pudding, vanilla, canned 5 oz	10	220	33
DAIRY	Pudding, vnlla,cooked from mix1/2 cup	4	145	25
DAIRY	Pudding, vnlla,instant frm mix1/2 cup	4	150	27
DAIRY	Quiche lorraine 1 slice	48	600	29
DAIRY	Ricotta cheese, part skim milk1 cup	19	340	13
DAIRY	Ricotta cheese, whole milk 1 cup	32	430	7
DAIRY	Shakes, thick, chocolate 10 oz	8	335	60
DAIRY	Shakes, thick, vanilla 10 oz	9	315	50
DAIRY	Sour cream 1 cup	48	495	10
DAIRY	Sour cream 1 tbsp	3	25	1
DAIRY	Swiss cheese 1 oz	8	105	1
DAIRY	Tofu 1 piece	5	85	3
DAIRY	Whipped topping, pressurized 1 cup	13	155	7
DAIRY	Whipped topping, pressurized 1 tbsp	1	10	0
DAIRY	Whipping cream, unwhiped,heavy1 cup	88	820	7
DAIRY	Whipping cream, unwhiped,heavy1 tbsp	6	50	0
DAIRY	Whipping cream, unwhiped,light1 cup	74	700	7
DAIRY	Whipping cream, unwhiped,light1 tbsp	5	45	0
DAIRY	Yogurt, w/ lofat milk, plain 8 oz	4	145	16
DAIRY	Yogurt, w/ lofat milk,fruitflv8 oz	2	230	43
DAIRY	Yogurt, w/ nonfat milk 8 oz	0	125	17
DAIRY	Yogurt, w/ whole milk 8 oz	7	140	11
FISH	Clams, canned, drained 3 oz	2	85	2
FISH	Clams, raw 3 oz	1	65	2
FISH	Crabmeat, canned 1 cup	3	135	1
FISH	Fish sandwich, lge, w/o cheese1 sandwh	27	470	41
FISH	Fish sandwich, reg, w/ cheese 1 sandwh	23	420	39
FISH	Fish sticks, frozen, reheated 1 stick	3	70	4
FISH	Flounder or sole, baked, buttr3 oz	6	120	0
FISH	Flounder or sole, baked,margrn3 oz	6	120	0
FISH	Flounder or sole, baked,w/ofat3 oz	1	80	0
FISH	Haddock, breaded, fried 3 oz	9	175	7

CHART BY FOOD CATEGORY

		Fat Grams	Food Energy Calories	Carbohydrate Grams
FISH	Halibut, broiled, butter,lemju3 oz	6	140	0
FISH	Herring, pickled 3 oz	13	190	0
FISH	Ocean perch, breaded, fried 1 fillet	11	185	7
FISH	Oysters, breaded, fried 1 oyster	5	90	5
FISH	Oysters, raw 1 cup	4	160	8
FISH	Salmon, baked, red 3 oz	5	140	0
FISH	Salmon, canned, pink, w/ bones3 oz	5	120	0
FISH	Salmon, smoked 3 oz	8	150	0
FISH	Sardines, atlntc,cnned,oil,drn3 oz	9	175	0
FISH	Scallops, breaded, frzn,reheat6 scalop	10	195	10
FISH	Shrimp, canned, drained 3 oz	1	100	1
FISH	Shrimp, french fried 3 oz	10	200	11
FISH	Trout, broiled, w/ buttr,lemju3 oz	9	175	0
FISH	Tuna salad 1 cup	19	375	19
FISH	Tuna, cannd, drnd,oil,chk,lght3 oz	7	165	0
FISH	Tuna, cannd, drnd,watr, white 3 oz	1	135	0
FRUITS	Apples, dried, sulfured 10 rings	0	155	42
FRUITS	Apples, raw, peeled, sliced 1 cup	0	65	16
FRUITS	Apples, raw, unpeeled,2 per lb1 apple	1	125	32
FRUITS	Apples, raw, unpeeled,3 per lb1 apple	0	80	21
FRUITS	Applesauce, canned, sweetened 1 cup	0	195	51
FRUITS	Applesauce, canned,unsweetened1 cup	0	105	28
FRUITS	Apricot nectar, no added vit c1 cup	0	140	36
FRUITS	Apricot, canned, heavy syrup 1 cup	0	215	55
FRUITS	Apricot, canned, heavy syrup 3 halves	0	70	18
FRUITS	Apricots, canned, juice pack 1 cup	0	120	31
FRUITS	Apricots, canned, juice pack 3 halves	0	40	10
FRUITS	Apricots, dried, cooked,unswtn1 cup	0	210	55
FRUITS	Apricots, dried, uncooked 1 cup	1	310	80
FRUITS	Apricots, raw 3 aprcot	0	50	12
FRUITS	Bananas 1 banana	1	105	27
FRUITS	Bananas, sliced 1 cup	1	140	35
FRUITS	Blackberries, raw 1 cup	1	75	18
FRUITS	Blueberries, frozen, sweetened1 cup	0	185	50
FRUITS	Blueberries, frozen, sweetened10 oz	0	230	62
FRUITS	Blueberries, raw 1 cup	1	80	20
FRUITS	Cantaloup, raw 1/2 meln	1	95	22
FRUITS	Cherries, sour,red,cannd,water1 cup	0	90	22
FRUITS	Cherries, sweet, raw 10 chery	1	50	11
FRUITS	Honeydew melon, raw 1/10 mel	0	45	12
FRUITS	Jams and preserves 1 pkt	0	40	10

CHART BY FOOD CATEGORY

			Fat Grams	Food Energy Calories	Carbohydrate Grams
FRUITS	Jams and preserves	1 tbsp	0	55	14
FRUITS	Jellies	1 pkt	0	40	10
FRUITS	Jellies	1 tbsp	0	50	13
FRUITS	Kiwifruit, raw	1 kiwi	0	45	11
FRUITS	Lemon juice, canned	1 cup	1	50	16
FRUITS	Lemon juice, canned	1 tbsp	0	5	1
FRUITS	Lemon juice, raw	1 cup	0	60	21
FRUITS	Lemons, raw	1 lemon	0	15	5
FRUITS	Plantains, cooked	1 cup	0	180	48
FRUITS	Plantains, raw	1 plantn	1	220	57
FRUITS	Plums, canned, heavy syrup	1 cup	0	230	60
FRUITS	Plums, canned, heavy syrup	3 plums	0	120	31
FRUITS	Plums, canned, juice pack	1 cup	0	145	38
FRUITS	Plums, canned, juice pack	3 plums	0	55	14
FRUITS	Plums, raw, 1-1/2-in diam	1 plum	0	15	4
FRUITS	Plums, raw, 2-1/8-in diam	1 plum	0	35	9
FRUITS	Prune juice, canned	1 cup	0	180	45
FRUITS	Prunes, dried	5 large	0	115	31
FRUITS	Prunes, dried, cooked,unswtned	1 cup	0	225	60
FRUITS	Raisins	1 cup	1	435	115
FRUITS	Raisins	1 packet	0	40	11
FRUITS	Raspberries, frozen, sweetened	1 cup	0	255	65
FRUITS	Raspberries, frozen, sweetened	10 oz	0	295	74
FRUITS	Raspberries, raw	1 cup	1	60	14
FRUITS	Rhubarb, cooked, added sugar	1 cup	0	280	75
FRUITS	Strawberries, frozen, sweetend	1 cup	0	245	66
FRUITS	Strawberries, frozen, sweetend	10 oz	0	275	74
FRUITS	Strawberries, raw	1 cup	1	45	10
FRUITS	Tangerine juice, canned,swtned	1 cup	0	125	30
FRUITS	Tangerines, canned, light syrp	1 cup	0	155	41
FRUITS	Tangerines, raw	1 tangrn	0	35	9
FRUITS	Watermelon, raw	1 piece	2	155	35
FRUITS	Watermelon, raw, diced	1 cup	1	50	11
FRUITS	Cranberry sauce, canned,swtnd	1 cup	0	420	108
FRUITS	Figs, dried	10 figs	2	475	122
FRUITS	Fruit cocktail,cnnd,heavysyrup	1 cup	0	185	48
FRUITS	Fruit cocktail,cnnd,juice pack	1 cup	0	115	29
FRUITS	Grapes, european, raw, thompsn	10 grape	0	35	9
FRUITS	Grapes, european, raw, tokay	10 grape	0	40	10
FRUITS	Lime juice, raw	1 cup	0	65	22
FRUITS	Lime juice,canned	1 cup	1	50	16

CHART BY FOOD CATEGORY

			Fat Grams	Food Energy Calories	Carbohydrate Grams
FRUITS	Nectarines, raw	1 nectrn	1	65	16
FRUITS	Oranges, raw	1 orange	0	60	15
FRUITS	Oranges, raw, sections	1 cup	0	85	21
FRUITS	Papayas, raw	1 cup	0	65	17
FRUITS	Peaches, canned, heavy syrup	1 cup	0	190	51
FRUITS	Peaches, canned, heavy syrup	1 half	0	60	16
FRUITS	Peaches, canned, juice pack	1 cup	0	110	29
FRUITS	Peaches, canned, juice pack	1 half	0	35	9
FRUITS	Peaches, dried	1 cup	1	380	98
FRUITS	Peaches, dried,cooked,unswetnd	1 cup	1	200	51
FRUITS	Peaches, frozen,swetned,w/vitc	1 cup	0	235	60
FRUITS	Peaches, frozen,swetned,w/vitc	10 oz	0	265	68
FRUITS	Peaches, raw	1 peach	0	35	10
FRUITS	Peaches, raw, sliced	1 cup	0	75	19
FRUITS	Pears, canned, heavy syrup	1 cup	0	190	49
FRUITS	Pears, canned, heavy syrup	1 half	0	60	15
FRUITS	Pears, canned, juice pack	1 cup	0	125	32
FRUITS	Pears, canned, juice pack	1 half	0	40	10
FRUITS	Pears, raw, bartlett	1 pear	1	100	25
FRUITS	Pears, raw, bosc	1 pear	1	85	21
FRUITS	Pears, raw, d'anjou	1 pear	1	120	30
FRUITS	Pineapple, canned, heavy syrup	1 cup	0	200	52
FRUITS	Pineapple, canned, heavy syrup	1 slice	0	45	12
FRUITS	Pineapple, canned, juice pack	1 cup	0	150	39
FRUITS	Pineapple, canned, juice pack	1 slice	0	35	9
FRUITS	Pineapple, raw, diced	1 cup	1	75	19
MEATS	Beef and vegetable stew,hm rcp	1 cup	11	220	15
MEATS	Beef heart, braised	3 oz	5	150	0
MEATS	Beef liver, fried	3 oz	7	185	7
MEATS	Beef potpie, home recipe	1 piece	30	515	39
MEATS	Beef roast, eye o rnd, lean	2.6 oz	5	135	0
MEATS	Beef roast, eye o rnd,lean+fat	3 oz	12	205	0
MEATS	Beef roast, rib, lean + fat	3 oz	26	315	0
MEATS	Beef roast, rib, lean only	2.2 oz	9	150	0
MEATS	Beef steak,sirloin,broil,lean	2.5 oz	6	150	0
MEATS	Beef steak,sirloin,broil,ln+ft	3 oz	15	240	0
MEATS	Beef, canned, corned	3 oz	10	185	0
MEATS	Beef, ckd,bttm round,lean only	2.8 oz	8	175	0
MEATS	Beef, ckd,bttm round,lean+ fat	3 oz	13	220	0
MEATS	Beef, ckd,chuck blade,lean+fat	3 oz	26	325	0
MEATS	Beef, ckd,chuck blade,leanonly	2.2 oz	9	170	0

CHART BY FOOD CATEGORY

			Fat Grams	Food Energy Calories	Carbohydrate Grams
MEATS	Beef, dried, chipped	2.5 oz	4	145	0
MEATS	Bologna	2 slices	16	180	2
MEATS	Braunschweiger	2 slices	18	205	2
MEATS	Brown and serve sausage,brwnd 1 link		5	50	0
MEATS	Cheeseburger, 4oz patty	1 sandwh	31	525	40
MEATS	Cheeseburger, regular	1 sandwh	15	300	28
MEATS	Chop suey w/ beef + pork,hmrcp1 cup		17	300	13
MEATS	Frankfurter, cooked	1 frank	13	145	1
MEATS	Ground beef, broiled, lean	3 oz	16	230	0
MEATS	Ground beef, broiled, regular 3 oz		18	245	0
MEATS	Hamburger, 4oz patty	1 sandwh	21	445	38
MEATS	Hamburger, regular	1 sandwh	11	245	28
MEATS	Lamb, rib, roasted, lean + fat3 oz		26	315	0
MEATS	Lamb, rib, roasted, lean only 2 oz		7	130	0
MEATS	Lamb,chops,arm,braised,lean 1.7 oz		7	135	0
MEATS	Lamb,chops,arm,braised,lean+ft2.2 oz		15	220	0
MEATS	Lamb,chops,loin,broil,lean 2.3 oz		6	140	0
MEATS	Lamb,chops,loin,broil,lean+fat2.8 oz		16	235	0
MEATS	Lamb,leg,roasted, lean only 2.6 oz		6	140	0
MEATS	Lamb,leg,roasted, lean+ fat 3 oz		13	205	0
MEATS	Pork chop, loin, broil, lean 2.5 oz		8	165	0
MEATS	Pork chop, loin, broil, len+ft3.1 oz		19	275	0
MEATS	Pork chop, loin,panfry, lean 2.4 oz		11	180	0
MEATS	Pork chop, loin,panfry,lean+ft3.1 oz		27	335	0
MEATS	Pork fresh ham, roastd, lean 2.5 oz		8	160	0
MEATS	Pork fresh ham, roastd,lean+ft3 oz		18	250	0
MEATS	Pork fresh rib, roastd, lean 2.5 oz		10	175	0
MEATS	Pork fresh rib, roastd,lean+ft3 oz		20	270	0
MEATS	Pork shoulder, braisd, lean 2.4 oz		8	165	0
MEATS	Pork shoulder, braisd,lean+fat3 oz		22	295	0
MEATS	Pork, cured, bacon, regul,cked3 slice		9	110	0
MEATS	Pork, cured, bacon,canadn,cked2 slice		4	85	1
MEATS	Pork, cured, ham, canned,roast3 oz		7	140	0
MEATS	Pork, cured, ham, rosted,lean 2.4 oz		4	105	0
MEATS	Pork, cured, ham, rosted,ln+ft3 oz		14	205	0
MEATS	Pork, link, cooked	1 link	4	50	0
MEATS	Pork, luncheon meat,canned	2 slices	13	140	1
MEATS	Pork, luncheon meat,choppd ham2 slices		7	95	0
MEATS	Pork, luncheon meat,ckd ham,ln2 slices		3	75	1
MEATS	Pork, luncheon meat,ckd ham,rg2 slices		6	105	2
MEATS	Roast beef sandwich	1 sandwh	13	345	34

CHART BY FOOD CATEGORY

			Fat Grams	Food Energy Calories	Carbohydrate Grams
MEATS	Salami, cooked type	2 slices	11	145	1
MEATS	Salami, dry type	2 slices	7	85	1
MEATS	Veal cutlet, med fat,brsd,brld	3 oz	9	185	0
MEATS	Veal rib, med fat, roasted	3 oz	14	230	0
MEATS	Vienna sausage	1 sausag	4	45	0
NUTS	Almonds, slivered	1 cup	70	795	28
NUTS	Almonds, whole	1 oz	15	165	6
NUTS	Brazil nuts	1 oz	19	185	4
NUTS	Cashew nuts, dry roastd,salted	1 oz	13	165	9
NUTS	Cashew nuts, dry roastd,unsalt	1 cup	63	785	45
NUTS	Cashew nuts, dry roastd,unsalt	1 oz	13	165	9
NUTS	Cashew nuts, dry roasted,saltd	1 cup	63	785	45
NUTS	Cashew nuts, oil roastd,salted	1 cup	63	750	37
NUTS	Cashew nuts, oil roastd,salted	1 oz	14	165	8
NUTS	Cashew nuts, oil roastd,unsalt	1 cup	63	750	37
NUTS	Cashew nuts, oil roastd,unsalt	1 oz	14	165	8
NUTS	Chestnuts, european, roasted	1 cup	3	350	76
NUTS	Dates	10 dates	0	230	61
NUTS	Dates, chopped	1 cup	1	490	131
NUTS	Filberts, (hazelnuts) chopped	1 cup	72	725	18
NUTS	Filberts, (hazelnuts) chopped	1 oz	18	180	4
NUTS	Macadamia nuts, oilrstd,salted	1 cup	103	960	17
NUTS	Macadamia nuts, oilrstd,salted	1 oz	22	205	4
NUTS	Macadamia nuts, oilrstd,unsalt	1 cup	103	960	17
NUTS	Macadamia nuts, oilrstd,unsalt	1 oz	22	205	4
NUTS	Mixed nuts w/ peants,dry,saltd	1 oz	15	170	7
NUTS	Mixed nuts w/ peants,dry,unslt	1 oz	15	170	7
NUTS	Mixed nuts w/ peants,oil,saltd	1 oz	16	175	6
NUTS	Mixed nuts w/ peants,oil,unslt	1 oz	16	175	6
NUTS	Peanut butter	1 tbsp	8	95	3
NUTS	Peanut butter cookie,home recp	4 cookie	14	245	28
NUTS	Peanuts, oil roasted, salted	1 cup	71	840	27
NUTS	Peanuts, oil roasted, salted	1 oz	14	165	5
NUTS	Peanuts, oil roasted, unsalted	1 cup	71	840	27
NUTS	Peanuts, oil roasted, unsalted	1 oz	14	165	5
NUTS	Pecans, halves	1 cup	73	720	20
NUTS	Pecans, halves	1 oz	19	190	5
NUTS	Pine nuts	1 oz	17	160	5
NUTS	Pistachio nuts	1 oz	14	165	7
NUTS	Popcorn, air-popped, unsalted	1 cup	0	30	6
NUTS	Popcorn, popped, veg oil,saltd	1 cup	3	55	6

CHART BY FOOD CATEGORY

		Fat Grams	Food Energy Calories	Carbohydrate Grams
NUTS	Popcorn, sugar syrup coated 1 cup	1	135	30
NUTS	Sunflower seeds 1 oz	14	160	5
NUTS	Walnuts, black, chopped 1 cup	71	760	15
NUTS	Walnuts, black, chopped 1 oz	16	170	3
NUTS	Walnuts, english, pieces 1 cup	74	770	22
NUTS	Walnuts, english, pieces 1 oz	18	180	5
NUTS	Water chestnuts, canned 1 cup	0	70	17
OILS	Safflower oil 1 cup	218	1925	0
OILS	Safflower oil 1 tbsp	14	125	0
OILS	Sunflower oil 1 cup	218	1925	0
OILS	Sunflower oil 1 tbsp	14	125	0
PASTA	Bulgur, uncooked 1 cup	3	600	129
PASTA	Macaroni and cheese, canned 1 cup	10	230	26
PASTA	Macaroni and cheese, home rcpe1 cup	22	430	40
PASTA	Macaroni, cooked, firm 1 cup	1	190	39
PASTA	Macaroni, cooked, tender, hot 1 cup	1	155	32
PASTA	Macaroni, cooked, tender,cold 1 cup	0	115	24
PASTA	Noodles, chow mein, canned 1 cup	11	220	26
PASTA	Noodles, egg, cooked 1 cup	2	200	37
PASTA	Spaghetti, cooked, firm 1 cup	1	190	39
PASTA	Spaghetti, cooked, tender 1 cup	1	155	32
PASTA	Spaghetti, tom sauce chee,hmrp1 cup	9	260	37
PASTA	Spaghetti, tom sauce chees,cnd1 cup	2	190	39
PASTA	Spaghetti,meatballs,tomsa,hmrp1 cup	12	330	39
PASTA	Spaghetti,meatballs,tomsac,cnd1 cup	10	260	29
POULTRY	Chicken a la king, home recipe1 cup	34	470	12
POULTRY	Chicken and noodles, home recp1 cup	18	365	26
POULTRY	Chicken chow mein, canned 1 cup	0	95	18
POULTRY	Chicken chow mein, home recipe1 cup	10	255	10
POULTRY	Chicken frankfurter 1 frank	9	115	3
POULTRY	Chicken liver, cooked 1 liver	1	30	0
POULTRY	Chicken potpie, home recipe 1 piece	31	545	42
POULTRY	Chicken roll, light 2 slices	4	90	1
POULTRY	Chicken, canned, boneless 5 oz	11	235	0
POULTRY	Chicken, fried, batter, breast4.9 oz	18	365	13
POULTRY	Chicken, fried, batter,drmstck2.5 oz	11	195	6
POULTRY	Chicken, fried, flour, breast 3.5 oz	9	220	2
POULTRY	Chicken, fried, flour, drmstck1.7 oz	7	120	1
POULTRY	Chicken, roasted, breast 3.0 oz	3	140	0
POULTRY	Chicken, roasted, drumstick 1.6 oz	2	75	0
POULTRY	Chicken, stewed, light + dark 1 cup	9	250	0

CHART BY FOOD CATEGORY

		Fat Grams	Food Energy Calories	Carbohydrate Grams
POULTRY	Duck, roasted, flesh only 1/2 duck	25	445	0
POULTRY	Turkey ham, cured turkey thigh2 slices	3	75	0
POULTRY	Turkey loaf, breast meat w/o c2 slices	1	45	0
POULTRY	Turkey loaf, breast meat, w/ c2 slices	1	45	0
POULTRY	Turkey patties, brd,battd,frid1 patty	12	180	10
POULTRY	Turkey roast, frzn,lght+drk,ck3 oz	5	130	3
POULTRY	Turkey, roasted, dark meat 4 pieces	6	160	0
POULTRY	Turkey, roasted, light + dark 1 cup	7	240	0
POULTRY	Turkey, roasted, light + dark 3 pieces	4	145	0
POULTRY	Turkey, roasted, light meat 2 pieces	3	135	0
RICE	Rice, brown, cooked 1 cup	1	230	50
RICE	Rice, white, cooked 1 cup	0	225	50
RICE	Rice, white, instant, cooked 1 cup	0	180	40
RICE	Rice, white, parboiled, cooked1 cup	0	185	41
RICE	Rice, white, parboiled, raw 1 cup	1	685	150
RICE	Rice, white, raw 1 cup	1	670	149
SAUCES	1000 island, salad drsng,local1 tbsp	2	25	2
SAUCES	1000 island, salad drsng,reglr1 tbsp	6	60	2
SAUCES	Barbecue sauce 1 tbsp	0	10	2
SAUCES	Beef gravy, canned 1 cup	5	125	11
SAUCES	Blue cheese salad dressing 1 tbsp	8	75	1
SAUCES	Brown gravy from dry mix 1 cup	2	80	14
SAUCES	Catsup 1 cup	1	290	69
SAUCES	Catsup 1 tbsp	0	15	4
SAUCES	Chicken gravy from dry mix 1 cup	2	85	14
SAUCES	Chicken gravy, canned 1 cup	14	190	13
SAUCES	Cooked salad drssing, home rcp1 tbsp	2	25	2
SAUCES	Corn oil 1 cup	218	1925	0
SAUCES	Corn oil 1 tbsp	14	125	0
SAUCES	Fats, cooking/vegetbl shorteng1 cup	205	1810	0
SAUCES	Fats, cooking/vegetbl shorteng1 tbsp	13	115	0
SAUCES	French salad dressing, localor1 tbsp	2	25	2
SAUCES	French salad dressing, regular1 tbsp	9	85	1
SAUCES	Gravy and turkey, frozen 5 oz	4	95	7
SAUCES	Hollandaise sce, w/ h2o,frm mx1 cup	20	240	14
SAUCES	Italian salad dressing,localor1 tbsp	0	5	2
SAUCES	Italian salad dressing,regular1 tbsp	9	80	1
SAUCES	Mayonnaise type salad dressing1 tbsp	5	60	4
SAUCES	Mayonnaise, imitation 1 tbsp	3	35	2
SAUCES	Mayonnaise, regular 1 tbsp	11	100	0
SAUCES	Mushroom gravy, canned 1 cup	6	120	13

CHART BY FOOD CATEGORY

			Fat Grams	Food Energy Calories	Carbohydrate Grams
SAUCES	Mustard, prepared, yellow	1 tsp	0	5	0
SAUCES	Olive oil	1 cup	216	1910	0
SAUCES	Olive oil	1 tbsp	14	125	0
SAUCES	Peanut oil	1 cup	216	1910	0
SAUCES	Peanut oil	1 tbsp	14	125	0
SAUCES	Soy sauce	1 tbsp	0	10	2
SAUCES	Soybean oil, hydrogenated	1 cup	218	1925	0
SAUCES	Soybean oil, hydrogenated	1 tbsp	14	125	0
SAUCES	Soybean-cottonseed oil, hydrgn	1 cup	218	1925	0
SAUCES	Soybean-cottonseed oil, hydrgn	1 tbsp	14	125	0
SAUCES	Soybeans, dry, cooked, drained	1 cup	10	235	19
SAUCES	Tartar sauce	1 tbsp	8	75	1
SAUCES	Tomato paste, canned w/o salt	1 cup	2	220	49
SAUCES	Tomato paste, canned with salt	1 cup	2	220	49
SAUCES	Tomato puree, canned w/o salt	1 cup	0	105	25
SAUCES	Tomato puree, canned with salt	1 cup	0	105	25
SAUCES	Tomato sauce, canned with salt	1 cup	0	75	18
SAUCES	Vinegar and oil salad dressing	1 tbsp	8	70	0
SAUCES	Vinegar, cider	1 tbsp	0	0	1
SOUPS	Beef broth, boulln, consm,cnnd	1 cup	1	15	0
SOUPS	Beef noodle soup, canned	1 cup	3	85	9
SOUPS	Bouillon, dehydrtd, unprepared	1 pkt	1	15	1
SOUPS	Chicken noodle soup, canned	1 cup	2	75	9
SOUPS	Chicken noodle soup,dehyd,prpd	1 pkt	1	40	6
SOUPS	Chicken rice soup, canned	1 cup	2	60	7
SOUPS	Clam chowder, manhattan, cannd	1 cup	2	80	12
SOUPS	Clam chowder, new eng, w/ milk	1 cup	7	165	17
SOUPS	Cr of chicken soup w/ h20,cnnd	1 cup	7	115	9
SOUPS	Cr of chicken soup w/ mlk,cnnd	1 cup	11	190	15
SOUPS	Cr of mushrom soup w/ h2o,cnnd	1 cup	9	130	9
SOUPS	Cr of mushrom soup w/ mlk,cnnd	1 cup	14	205	15
SOUPS	Minestrone soup, canned	1 cup	3	80	11
SOUPS	Onion soup, dehydratd, prepred	1 pkt	0	20	4
SOUPS	Onion soup, dehydrtd, unprpred	1 pkt	0	20	4
SOUPS	Pea, green, soup, canned	1 cup	3	165	27
SOUPS	Tomato soup w/ water, canned	1 cup	2	85	17
SOUPS	Tomato soup with milk, canned	1 cup	6	160	22
SOUPS	Tomato veg soup, dehyd,prepred	1 pkt	1	40	8
SOUPS	Vegetable beef soup, canned	1 cup	2	80	10
SOUPS	Vegetarian soup, canned	1 cup	2	70	12
SPICES	Celery seed	1 tsp	1	10	1

CHART BY FOOD CATEGORY

			Fat Grams	Food Energy Calories	Carbohydrate Grams
SPICES	Chili powder	1 tsp	0	10	1
SPICES	Cinnamon	1 tsp	0	5	2
SPICES	Curry powder	1 tsp	0	5	1
SPICES	Garlic powder	1 tsp	0	10	2
SPICES	Onion powder	1 tsp	0	5	2
SPICES	Oregano	1 tsp	0	5	1
SPICES	Paprika	1 tsp	0	5	1
SPICES	Parsley, freeze-dried	1 tbsp	0	0	0
SPICES	Pepper, black	1 tsp	0	5	1
SPICES	Salt	1 tsp	0	0	0
SPICES	Sesame seeds	1 tbsp	4	45	1
SWEETS	Angelfood cake, from mix	1 cake	2	1510	342
SWEETS	Angelfood cake, from mix	1 piece	0	125	29
SWEETS	Apple pie	1 pie	105	2420	360
SWEETS	Apple pie	1 piece	18	405	60
SWEETS	Blueberry muffins, home recipe	1 muffin	5	135	20
SWEETS	Blueberry muffins,from com mix	1 muffin	5	140	22
SWEETS	Blueberry pie	1 pie	102	2285	330
SWEETS	Blueberry pie	1 piece	17	380	55
SWEETS	Brownies w/ nuts,frm home recp	1 browne	6	95	11
SWEETS	Brownies w/ nuts,frstng,cmmrcl	1 browne	4	100	16
SWEETS	Caramels, plain or chocolate	1 oz	3	115	22
SWEETS	Carrot cake,cremchese frst,rec	1 cake	328	6175	775
SWEETS	Carrot cake,cremchese frst,rec	1 piece	21	385	48
SWEETS	Cheesecake	1 cake	213	3350	317
SWEETS	Cheesecake	1 piece	18	280	26
SWEETS	Cherry pie	1 pie	107	2465	363
SWEETS	Cherry pie	1 piece	18	410	61
SWEETS	Chocolate chip cookies,commrcl	4 cookie	9	180	28
SWEETS	Chocolate chip cookies,hme rcp	4 cookie	11	185	26
SWEETS	Chocolate chip cookies,refrig	4 cookie	11	225	32
SWEETS	Chocolate, bitter ot baking	1 oz	15	145	8
SWEETS	Coca pwdr w/o nofat drymlk,prd	1 servng	9	225	30
SWEETS	Coca pwdr w/o nonfat dry milk	3/4 oz	1	75	19
SWEETS	Cocoa pwdr w/ nofat drmlk,prpd	1 servng	1	100	22
SWEETS	Cocoa pwdr with nonfat drymilk	1 oz	1	100	22
SWEETS	Coconut, dried, sweetnd,shredd	1 cup	33	470	44
SWEETS	Coconut, raw, piece	1 piece	15	160	7
SWEETS	Coconut, raw, shredded	1 cup	27	285	12
SWEETS	Creme pie	1 pie	139	2710	351
SWEETS	Creme pie	1 piece	23	455	59

CHART BY FOOD CATEGORY

			Fat Grams	Food Energy Calories	Carbohydrate Grams
SWEETS	Custard pie	1 pie	101	1985	213
SWEETS	Custard pie	1 piece	17	330	36
SWEETS	Custard, baked	1 cup	15	305	29
SWEETS	Devil's food cake,chocfrst,fmx1 cake		136	3755	645
SWEETS	Devil's food cake,chocfrst,fmx1 cupcak		4	120	20
SWEETS	Devil's food cake,chocfrst,fmx1 piece		8	235	40
SWEETS	Doughnuts, cake type, plain	1 donut	12	210	24
SWEETS	Doughnuts, yeast-leavend,glzed1 donut		13	235	26
SWEETS	Fig bars	4 cookie	4	210	42
SWEETS	Fried pie, apple	1 pie	14	255	31
SWEETS	Fried pie, cherry	1 pie	14	250	32
SWEETS	Fruitcake,dark, from homerecip1 cake		228	5185	783
SWEETS	Fruitcake,dark, from homerecip1 piece		7	165	25
SWEETS	Fudge, chocolate, plain	1 oz	3	115	21
SWEETS	Gingerbread cake, from mix	1 cake	39	1575	291
SWEETS	Gingerbread cake, from mix	1 piece	4	175	32
SWEETS	Graham cracker, plain	2 crackr	1	60	11
SWEETS	Gum drops	1 oz	0	100	25
SWEETS	Hard candy	1 oz	0	110	28
SWEETS	Honey	1 cup	0	1030	279
SWEETS	Honey	1 tbsp	0	65	17
SWEETS	Jelly beans	1 oz	0	105	26
SWEETS	Lemon meringue pie	1 pie	86	2140	317
SWEETS	Lemon meringue pie	1 piece	14	355	53
SWEETS	Marshmallows	1 oz	0	90	23
SWEETS	Milk chocolate candy, plain	1 oz	9	145	16
SWEETS	Milk chocolate candy,w/ almond1 oz		10	150	15
SWEETS	Milk chocolate candy,w/ penuts1 oz		11	155	13
SWEETS	Milk chocolate candy,w/ rice c1 oz		7	140	18
SWEETS	Molasses, cane, blackstrap	2 tbsp	0	85	22
SWEETS	Peach pie	1 pie	101	2410	361
SWEETS	Peach pie	1 piece	17	405	60
SWEETS	Pecan pie	1 pie	189	3450	423
SWEETS	Pecan pie	1 piece	32	575	71
SWEETS	Popsicle	1 popcle	0	170	18
SWEETS	Pound cake, commercial	1 loaf	94	1935	257
SWEETS	Pound cake, commercial	1 slice	5	110	15
SWEETS	Pound cake, from home recipe	1 loaf	94	2025	265
SWEETS	Pound cake, from home recipe	1 slice	5	120	15
SWEETS	Pumpkin pie	1 pie	102	1920	223
SWEETS	Pumpkin pie	1 piece	17	320	37

CHART BY FOOD CATEGORY

			Fat Grams	Food Energy Calories	Carbohydrate Grams
SWEETS	Sandwich type cookie	4 cookie	8	195	29
SWEETS	Semisweet chocolate	1 cup	61	860	97
SWEETS	Sheetcake w/o frstng,homerecip	1 cake	108	2830	434
SWEETS	Sheetcake,w/ whfrstng,homercip	1 cake	129	4020	694
SWEETS	Sheetcake,w/ whfrstng,homercip	1 piece	14	445	77
SWEETS	Sheetcake,w/o frstng,homerecip	1 piece	12	315	48
SWEETS	Sherbet, 2% fat	1 cup	4	270	59
SWEETS	Sherbet, 2% fat	1/2 gal	31	2160	469
SWEETS	Shortbread cookie, commercial	4 cookie	8	1556	20
SWEETS	Shortbread cookie, home recipe	2 cookie	8	145	17
SWEETS	Snack cakes,devils food,cremflsm	cake	4	105	17
SWEETS	Snack cakes,sponge creme fllngsm	cake	5	155	27
SWEETS	Sugar cookie, from refrig dogh	4 cookie	12	235	31
SWEETS	Sugar, brown, pressed down	1 cup	0	820	212
SWEETS	Sugar, powdered, sifted	1 cup	0	385	100
SWEETS	Sugar, white, granulated	1 cup	0	770	199
SWEETS	Sugar, white, granulated	1 pkt	0	25	6
SWEETS	Sugar, white, granulated	1 tbsp	0	45	12
SWEETS	Sweet (dark) chocolate	1 oz	10	150	16
SWEETS	Sweetened condensed milk cnnd	1 cup	27	980	166
SWEETS	Syrup, chocolate flavored thin	2 tbsp	0	85	22
SWEETS	Syrup, chocolate flvred, fudge	2 tbsp	5	125	21
SWEETS	Table syrup (corn and maple)	2 tbsp	0	122	32
SWEETS	Vanilla wafers	10 cooke	7	185	29
SWEETS	White cake w/ wht frstng,comml	1 cake	148	4170	670
SWEETS	White cake w/ wht frstng,comml	1 piece	9	260	42
SWEETS	White sauce w/ milk from mix	1 cup	13	240	21
SWEETS	White sauce, medium, home recp	1 cup	30	395	24
SWEETS	Whole-wheat bread	1 loaf	20	1110	206
SWEETS	Whole-wheat bread	1 slice	1	70	13
SWEETS	Whole-wheat bread, toasted	1 slice	1	70	13
SWEETS	Whole-wheat flour,hrd wht,stir	1 cup	2	400	85
SWEETS	Whole-wheat wafers, crackers	2 crackr	2	35	5
SWEETS	Yellow cake w/ choc frst,frmix	1 cake	125	3735	638
SWEETS	Yellow cake w/ choc frst,frmix	1 piece	8	235	40
SWEETS	Yellowcake w/ chocfrstng,comml	1 cake	175	3895	620
SWEETS	Yellowcake w/ chocfrstng,comml	1 piece	11	245	39
VEGETABLES	Alfalfa seeds, sprouted, raw	1 cup	0	10	1
VEGETABLES	Artichokes, globe, cooked, drn	1 artchk	0	55	12
VEGETABLES	Asparagus, ckd frm frz,dr,sper	4 spears	0	15	3
VEGETABLES	Asparagus, ckd frm frz,drn,cut	1 cup	1	50	9

CHART BY FOOD CATEGORY

		Fat Grams	Food Energy Calories	Carbohydrate Grams
VEGETABLES	Asparagus, ckd frm raw, dr,cut1 cup	1	45	8
VEGETABLES	Asparagus, ckd frm raw,dr,sper4 spears	0	15	3
VEGETABLES	Asparagus,canned,spears,nosalt4 spears	0	10	2
VEGETABLES	Asparagus,canned,spears,w/salt4 spears	0	10	2
VEGETABLES	Avocados, california 1 avocdo	30	305	12
VEGETABLES	Avocados, florida 1 avocdo	27	340	27
VEGETABLES	Bamboo shoots, canned, drained1 cup	1	25	4
VEGETABLES	Barley, pearled,light, uncookd1 cup	2	700	158
VEGETABLES	Bean sprouts, mung, cookd,dran1 cup	0	25	5
VEGETABLES	Bean sprouts, mung, raw 1 cup	0	30	6
VEGETABLES	Bean with bacon soup, canned 1 cup	6	170	23
VEGETABLES	Beans,dry,canned,w/frankfurter1 cup	18	365	32
VEGETABLES	Beans,dry,canned,w/pork+swtsce1 cup	12	385	54
VEGETABLES	Beans,dry,canned,w/pork+tomsce1 cup	7	310	48
VEGETABLES	Beet greens, cooked, drained 1 cup	0	40	8
VEGETABLES	Beets, canned, drained,no salt1 cup	0	55	12
VEGETABLES	Beets, canned, drained,w/ salt1 cup	0	55	12
VEGETABLES	Beets, cooked, drained, diced 1 cup	0	55	11
VEGETABLES	Beets, cooked, drained, whole 2 beets	0	30	7
VEGETABLES	Black beans, dry, cooked,drand1 cup	1	225	41
VEGETABLES	Blackeye peas, immatr,raw,cked1 cup	1	180	30
VEGETABLES	Blackeye peas,immtr,frzn,cked 1 cup	1	225	40
VEGETABLES	Black-eyed peas, dry, cooked 1 cup	1	190	35
VEGETABLES	Broccoli, frzn, cooked, draned1 cup	0	50	10
VEGETABLES	Broccoli, frzn, cooked, draned1 piece	0	10	2
VEGETABLES	Broccoli, raw 1 spear	1	40	8
VEGETABLES	Broccoli, raw, cooked, drained1 cup	0	45	9
VEGETABLES	Broccoli, raw, cooked, drained1 spear	1	50	10
VEGETABLES	Brussels sprouts, frzn, cooked1 cup	1	65	13
VEGETABLES	Brussels sprouts, raw, cooked 1 cup	1	60	13
VEGETABLES	Cabbage, chinese, pak-choi,ckd1 cup	0	20	3
VEGETABLES	Cabbage, chinese,pe-tsai, raw 1 cup	0	10	2
VEGETABLES	Cabbage, common, cooked, drned1 cup	0	30	7
VEGETABLES	Cabbage, common, raw 1 cup	0	15	4
VEGETABLES	Cabbage, red, raw 1 cup	0	20	4
VEGETABLES	Cabbage, savoy, raw 1 cup	0	20	4
VEGETABLES	Carrots, canned, drn, w/ salt 1 cup	0	35	8
VEGETABLES	Carrots, canned,drnd, w/o salt1 cup	0	35	8
VEGETABLES	Carrots, cooked from frozen 1 cup	0	55	12
VEGETABLES	Carrots, cooked from raw 1 cup	0	70	16
VEGETABLES	Carrots, raw, grated 1 cup	0	45	11

CHART BY FOOD CATEGORY

		Fat Grams	Food Energy Calories	Carbohydrate Grams
VEGETABLES	Carrots, raw, whole 1 carrot	0	30	7
VEGETABLES	Cauliflower, cooked from frozn1 cup	0	35	7
VEGETABLES	Cauliflower, cooked from raw 1 cup	0	30	6
VEGETABLES	Cauliflower, raw 1 cup	0	25	5
VEGETABLES	Celery, pascal type, raw,piece1 cup	0	20	4
VEGETABLES	Celery, pascal type, raw,stalk1 stalk	0	5	1
VEGETABLES	Chickpeas, cooked, drained 1 cup	4	270	45
VEGETABLES	Chili con carne w/ beans, cnnd1 cup	16	340	31
VEGETABLES	Collards, cooked from frozen 1 cup	1	60	12
VEGETABLES	Collards, cooked from raw 1 cup	0	25	5
VEGETABLES	Corn, cnnd,crm stl,whit,no sal1 cup	1	185	46
VEGETABLES	Corn, cnnd,crm stl,whit,w/salt1 cup	1	185	46
VEGETABLES	Corn, cnnd,crm stl,yllw,no sal1 cup	1	185	46
VEGETABLES	Corn, cnnd,crm stl,yllw,w/salt1 cup	1	185	46
VEGETABLES	Corn, cooked frm frozn, white 1 cup	0	135	34
VEGETABLES	Corn, cooked frm frozn, white 1 ear	0	60	14
VEGETABLES	Corn, cooked frm frozn, yellow1 cup	0	135	34
VEGETABLES	Corn, cooked frm frozn, yellow1 ear	0	60	14
VEGETABLES	Corn, cooked from raw, white 1 ear	1	85	19
VEGETABLES	Corn, cooked from raw, yellow 1 ear	1	85	19
VEGETABLES	Corn,cnnd,whl krnl,whte,no sal1 cup	1	165	41
VEGETABLES	Corn,cnnd,whl krnl,whte,w/salt1 cup	1	165	41
VEGETABLES	Corn,cnnd,whl krnl,yllw,no sal1 cup	1	165	41
VEGETABLES	Corn,cnnd,whl krnl,yllw,w/salt1 cup	1	165	41
VEGETABLES	Cucumber, w/ peel 6 slices	0	5	1
VEGETABLES	Dandelion greens, cooked, drnd1 cup	1	35	7
VEGETABLES	Eggplant, cooked, steamed 1 cup	0	25	6
VEGETABLES	Endive, curly, raw 1 cup	0	10	2
VEGETABLES	Jerusalem-artichoke, raw 1 cup	0	115	26
VEGETABLES	Kale, cooked from frozen 1 cup	1	40	7
VEGETABLES	Kale, cooked from raw 1 cup	1	40	7
VEGETABLES	Lentils, dry, cooked 1 cup	1	215	38
VEGETABLES	Lettuce, butterhead, raw,head 1 head	0	20	4
VEGETABLES	Lettuce, butterhead, raw,leave1 leaf	0	0	0
VEGETABLES	Lettuce, crisphead, raw, head 1 head	1	70	11
VEGETABLES	Lettuce, crisphead, raw,pieces1 cup	0	5	1
VEGETABLES	Lettuce, crisphead, raw,wedge 1 wedge	0	20	3
VEGETABLES	Lettuce, looseleaf 1 cup	0	10	2
VEGETABLES	Lima beans, dry, cooked,draned1 cup	1	260	49
VEGETABLES	Lima beans,baby, frzn,cked,drn1 cup	1	190	35
VEGETABLES	Lima beans,thick seed,frzn,ckd1 cup	1	170	32

CHART BY FOOD CATEGORY

			Fat Grams	Food Energy Calories	Carbohydrate Grams
VEGETABLES	Mangos, raw	1 mango	1	135	35
VEGETABLES	Mushrooms, canned, drnd,w/salt	1 cup	0	35	8
VEGETABLES	Mushrooms, cooked, drained	1 cup	1	40	8
VEGETABLES	Mushrooms, raw	1 cup	0	20	3
VEGETABLES	Mustard greens, cooked, draned	1 cup	0	20	3
VEGETABLES	Okra pods, cooked	8 pods	0	25	6
VEGETABLES	Olives, canned, green	4 medium	2	15	0
VEGETABLES	Olives, canned, ripe, mission	3 small	2	15	0
VEGETABLES	Onion rings, breaded,frzn,prpd	2 rings	5	80	8
VEGETABLES	Onions, raw, chopped	1 cup	0	55	12
VEGETABLES	Onions, raw, cooked, drained	1 cup	0	60	13
VEGETABLES	Onions, raw, sliced	1 cup	0	40	8
VEGETABLES	Onions, spring, raw	6 onion	0	10	2
VEGETABLES	Orange soda	12 fl oz	0	180	46
VEGETABLES	Parsley, raw	10 sprig	0	5	1
VEGETABLES	Parsnips, cooked, drained	1 cup	0	125	30
VEGETABLES	Pea beans, dry, cooked,drained	1 cup	1	225	40
VEGETABLES	Peas, edible pod, cooked,drned	1 cup	0	65	11
VEGETABLES	Peas, green,cnnd,drnd, w/ salt	1 cup	1	115	21
VEGETABLES	Peas, green,cnnd,drnd,w/o salt	1 cup	1	115	21
VEGETABLES	Peas, split, dry, cooked	1 cup	1	230	42
VEGETABLES	Peas,grn, frozen cooked,draned	1 cup	0	125	23
VEGETABLES	Peppers, hot chili, raw, green	1 pepper	0	20	4
VEGETABLES	Peppers, hot chili, raw, red	1 pepper	0	20	4
VEGETABLES	Peppers, sweet, cooked, green	1 pepper	0	15	3
VEGETABLES	Peppers, sweet, cooked, red	1 pepper	0	15	3
VEGETABLES	Peppers, sweet, raw, green	1 pepper	0	20	4
VEGETABLES	Peppers, sweet, raw, red	1 pepper	0	20	4
VEGETABLES	Pickles, cucumber, dill	1 pickle	0	5	1
VEGETABLES	Pickles, cucumber, fresh pack	2 slices	0	10	3
VEGETABLES	Pickles, cucumber, swt gherkin	1 pickle	0	20	5
VEGETABLES	Pinto beans,dry,cooked,drained	1 cup	1	265	49
VEGETABLES	Potato salad made w/ mayonnais	1 cup	21	360	28
VEGETABLES	Potatoes, au gratin, from mix	1 cup	10	230	31
VEGETABLES	Potatoes, au gratin, home recp	1 cup	19	325	28
VEGETABLES	Potatoes, baked flesh only	1 potato	0	145	34
VEGETABLES	Potatoes, baked with skin	1 potato	0	220	51
VEGETABLES	Potatoes, boiled, peeled after	1 potato	0	120	27
VEGETABLES	Potatoes, boiled, peeled befor	1 potato	0	115	27
VEGETABLES	Potatoes, hashed brown,fr frzn	1 cup	18	340	44
VEGETABLES	Potatoes, mashed,frm dehydrted	1 cup	12	235	32

CHART BY FOOD CATEGORY

		Fat Grams	Food Energy Calories	Carbohydrate Grams
VEGETABLES	Potatoes, mashed,recpe,mlk+mar1 cup	9	225	35
VEGETABLES	Potatoes, mashed,recpe,w/ milk1 cup	1	160	37
VEGETABLES	Potatoes, scalloped, from mix 1 cup	11	230	31
VEGETABLES	Potatoes, scalloped, home recp1 cup	9	210	26
VEGETABLES	Potatoes,french-frd,frzn,fried10 strip	8	160	20
VEGETABLES	Potatoes,french-frd,frzn,oven 10 strip	4	110	17
VEGETABLES	Pumpkin and squash kernels 1 oz	13	155	5
VEGETABLES	Pumpkin, canned 1 cup	1	85	20
VEGETABLES	Pumpkin, cooked from raw 1 cup	0	50	12
VEGETABLES	Radishes, raw 4 radish	0	5	1
VEGETABLES	Red kidney beans, dry, canned 1 cup	1	230	42
VEGETABLES	Refried beans, canned 1 cup	3	295	51
VEGETABLES	Sauerkraut, canned 1 cup	0	45	10
VEGETABLES	Seaweed, kelp, raw 1 oz	0	10	3
VEGETABLES	Seaweed, spirulina, dried 1 oz	2	80	7
VEGETABLES	Snap bean,cnnd,drnd,green,salt1 cup	0	25	6
VEGETABLES	Snap bean,cnnd,drnd,grn,nosalt1 cup	0	25	6
VEGETABLES	Snap bean,cnnd,drnd,yllw, salt1 cup	0	25	6
VEGETABLES	Snap bean,cnnd,drnd,yllw,nosal1 cup	0	25	6
VEGETABLES	Snap bean,frz,ckd,drnd,green 1 cup	0	35	8
VEGETABLES	Snap bean,frz,ckd,drnd,yellow 1 cup	0	35	8
VEGETABLES	Snap bean,raw,ckd,drnd,green 1 cup	0	45	10
VEGETABLES	Snap bean,raw,ckd,drnd,yellow 1 cup	0	45	10
VEGETABLES	Spinach souffle 1 cup	18	220	3
VEGETABLES	Spinach, canned, drnd,w/ salt 1 cup	1	50	7
VEGETABLES	Spinach, canned, drnd,w/o salt1 cup	1	50	7
VEGETABLES	Spinach, cooked fr frzen, drnd1 cup	0	55	10
VEGETABLES	Spinach, cooked from raw, drnd1 cup	0	40	7
VEGETABLES	Spinach, raw 1 cup	0	10	2
VEGETABLES	Squash, summer, cooked, draind1 cup	1	35	8
VEGETABLES	Squash, winter, baked 1 cup	1	80	18
VEGETABLES	Sweetpotatoes, baked, peeled 1 potato	0	115	28
VEGETABLES	Sweetpotatoes, boiled w/o peel1 potato	0	160	37
VEGETABLES	Sweetpotatoes, candied 1 piece	3	145	29
VEGETABLES	Sweetpotatoes, canned, mashed 1 cup	1	260	59
VEGETABLES	Sweetpotatoes, cnned, vac pack1 piece	0	35	8
VEGETABLES	Tomatoes, canned, s+l, w/ salt1 cup	1	50	10
VEGETABLES	Tomatoes, canned, s+l,w/o salt1 cup	1	50	10
VEGETABLES	Tomatoes, raw 1 tomato	0	25	5
VEGETABLES	Turnip greens, cked frm frozen1 cup	1	50	8
VEGETABLES	Turnip greens, cooked from raw1 cup	0	30	6

CHART BY FOOD CATEGORY

			Fat Grams	Food Energy Calories	Carbohydrate Grams
VEGETABLES	Turnips, cooked, diced	1 cup	0	30	8
VEGETABLES	Vegetables, mixed, canned	1 cup	0	75	15
VEGETABLES	Vegetables, mixed, cked fr frz	1 cup	0	105	24

CHART BY CALORIES

CHART BY CALORIES

	FOOD		Food Energy Calories
BEVERAGES	Club soda	12 fl oz	0
BEVERAGES	Coffee, brewed	6 fl oz	0
BEVERAGES	Coffee, instant, prepared	6 fl oz	0
BEVERAGES	Cola, diet, aspartame only	12 fl oz	0
BEVERAGES	Cola, diet, asprtame + sacchrn	12 fl oz	0
BEVERAGES	Cola, diet, saccharin only	12 fl oz	0
VEGETABLES	Lettuce, butterhead, raw,leave	1 leaf	0
SPICES	Parsley, freeze-dried	1 tbsp	0
SPICES	Salt	1 tsp	0
BEVERAGES	Tea, brewed	8 fl oz	0
BEVERAGES	Tea, instant,preprd,unsweetend	8 fl oz	0
SAUCES	Vinegar, cider	1 tbsp	0
MISCELLANEOUS	Baking powder, low sodium	1 tsp	5
MISCELLANEOUS	Baking powder, strght phosphat	1 tsp	5
MISCELLANEOUS	Baking powder,sas, ca po4	1 tsp	5
BREADS	Baking powder,sas,capo4+caso4	1 tsp	5
VEGETABLES	Celery, pascal type, raw,stalk	1 stalk	5
SPICES	Cinnamon	1 tsp	5
VEGETABLES	Cucumber, w/ peel	6 slices	5
SPICES	Curry powder	1 tsp	5
SAUCES	Italian salad dressing,localor	1 tbsp	5
FRUITS	Lemon juice, canned	1 tbsp	5
VEGETABLES	Lettuce, crisphead, raw,pieces	1 cup	5
SAUCES	Mustard, prepared, yellow	1 tsp	5
SPICES	Onion powder	1 tsp	5
SPICES	Oregano	1 tsp	5
SPICES	Paprika	1 tsp	5
VEGETABLES	Parsley, raw	10 sprig	5
SPICES	Pepper, black	1 tsp	5
VEGETABLES	Pickles, cucumber, dill	1 pickle	5
VEGETABLES	Radishes, raw	4 radish	5
VEGETABLES	Alfalfa seeds, sprouted, raw	1 cup	10
VEGETABLES	Asparagus,canned,spears,nosalt	4 spears	10
VEGETABLES	Asparagus,canned,spears,w/salt	4 spears	10
SAUCES	Barbecue sauce	1 tbsp	10
VEGETABLES	Broccoli, frzn, cooked, draned	1 piece	10
VEGETABLES	Cabbage, chinese,pe-tsai, raw	1 cup	10

CHART BY CALORIES

	FOOD		Food Energy Calories
SPICES	Chili powder	1 tsp	10
VEGETABLES	Endive, curly, raw	1 cup	10
SPICES	Garlic powder	1 tsp	10
DAIRY	Imitatn whipd toping,pwdrd,prp1 tbsp		10
VEGETABLES	Lettuce, looseleaf	1 cup	10
VEGETABLES	Onions, spring, raw	6 onion	10
VEGETABLES	Pickles, cucumber, fresh pack 2 slices		10
BREADS	Pretzels, stick	10 pretz	10
VEGETABLES	Seaweed, kelp, raw	1 oz	10
SAUCES	Soy sauce	1 tbsp	10
VEGETABLES	Spinach, raw	1 cup	10
SPICES	Celery seed	1 tsp	10
DAIRY	Imitation creamers, powdered	1 tsp	10
DAIRY	Imitatn whipd toping,pressrzd 1 tbsp		10
DAIRY	Whipped topping, pressurized	1 tbsp	10
VEGETABLES	Asparagus, ckd frm frz,dr,sper4 spears		15
VEGETABLES	Asparagus, ckd frm raw,dr,sper4 spears		15
VEGETABLES	Cabbage, common, raw	1 cup	15
SAUCES	Catsup	1 tbsp	15
DAIRY	Eggs, raw, white	1 white	15
FRUITS	Lemons, raw	1 lemon	15
VEGETABLES	Peppers, sweet, cooked, green 1 pepper		15
VEGETABLES	Peppers, sweet, cooked, red 1 pepper		15
FRUITS	Plums, raw, 1-1/2-in diam	1 plum	15
SOUPS	Beef broth, boulln, consm,cnnd1 cup		15
SOUPS	Bouillon, dehydrtd, unprepared1 pkt		15
DAIRY	Imitation whipped topping,frzn1 tbsp		15
BREADS	Snack type crackers	1 crackr	15
VEGETABLES	Olives, canned, green	4 medium	15
VEGETABLES	Olives, canned, ripe, mission 3 small		15
VEGETABLES	Cabbage, chinese, pak-choi,ckd1 cup		20
VEGETABLES	Cabbage, red, raw	1 cup	20
VEGETABLES	Cabbage, savoy, raw	1 cup	20
VEGETABLES	Celery, pascal type, raw,piece1 cup		20
VEGETABLES	Lettuce, butterhead, raw,head 1 head		20
VEGETABLES	Lettuce, crisphead, raw,wedge 1 wedge		20
BREADS	Melba toast, plain	1 piece	20
VEGETABLES	Mushrooms, raw	1 cup	20
VEGETABLES	Mustard greens, cooked, draned1 cup		20
SOUPS	Onion soup, dehydratd, prepred1 pkt		20
SOUPS	Onion soup, dehydrtd, unprpred1 pkt		20

CHART BY CALORIES

	FOOD	Food Energy Calories
VEGETABLES	Peppers, hot chili, raw, green1 pepper	20
VEGETABLES	Peppers, hot chili, raw, red 1 pepper	20
VEGETABLES	Peppers, sweet, raw, green 1 pepper	20
VEGETABLES	Peppers, sweet, raw, red 1 pepper	20
VEGETABLES	Pickles, cucumber, swt gherkin1 pickle	20
SAUCES	Relish, sweet 1 tbsp	20
MISCELLANEOUS	Yeast, bakers, dry, active 1 pkg	20
DAIRY	Imitation creamers, liquid frz1 tbsp	20
BEVERAGES	Half and half, cream 1 tbsp	20
DAIRY	Imitatn sour dressing 1 tbsp	20
VEGETABLES	Bean sprouts, mung, cookd,dran1 cup	25
VEGETABLES	Cauliflower, raw 1 cup	25
VEGETABLES	Collards, cooked from raw 1 cup	25
VEGETABLES	Eggplant, cooked, steamed 1 cup	25
MISCELLANEOUS	Gelatin, dry 1 envelp	25
VEGETABLES	Okra pods, cooked 8 pods	25
VEGETABLES	Snap bean,cnnd,drnd,green,salt1 cup	25
VEGETABLES	Snap bean,cnnd,drnd,grn,nosalt1 cup	25
VEGETABLES	Snap bean,cnnd,drnd,yllw, salt1 cup	25
VEGETABLES	Snap bean,cnnd,drnd,yllw,nosal1 cup	25
SWEETS	Sugar, white, granulated 1 pkt	25
VEGETABLES	Tomatoes, raw 1 tomato	25
MISCELLANEOUS	Yeast, brewers, dry 1 tbsp	25
VEGETABLES	Bamboo shoots, canned, drained1 cup	25
SAUCES	1000 island, salad drsng,local1 tbsp	25
SAUCES	Cooked salad drssing, home rcp1 tbsp	25
SAUCES	French salad dressing, localor1 tbsp	25
DAIRY	Parmesan cheese, grated 1 tbsp	25
DAIRY	Margarine, spread,hard,60% fat1 pat	25
DAIRY	Sour cream 1 tbsp	25
VEGETABLES	Bean sprouts, mung, raw 1 cup	30
VEGETABLES	Beets, cooked, drained, whole 2 beets	30
VEGETABLES	Cabbage, common, cooked, drned1 cup	30
VEGETABLES	Carrots, raw, whole 1 carrot	30
VEGETABLES	Cauliflower, cooked from raw 1 cup	30
NUTS	Popcorn, air-popped, unsalted 1 cup	30
VEGETABLES	Turnip greens, cooked from raw1 cup	30
VEGETABLES	Turnips, cooked, diced 1 cup	30
POULTRY	Chicken liver, cooked 1 liver	30
DAIRY	Light, coffee or table cream 1 tbsp	30
VEGETABLES	Carrots, canned, drn, w/ salt 1 cup	35

185

CHART BY CALORIES

	FOOD	Food Energy Calories
VEGETABLES	Carrots, canned,drnd, w/o salt1 cup	35
VEGETABLES	Cauliflower, cooked from frozn1 cup	35
FRUITS	Grapes, european, raw, thompsn10 grape	35
VEGETABLES	Mushrooms, canned, drnd,w/salt1 cup	35
FRUITS	Peaches, canned, juice pack 1 half	35
FRUITS	Peaches, raw 1 peach	35
FRUITS	Pineapple, canned, juice pack 1 slice	35
FRUITS	Plums, raw, 2-1/8-in diam 1 plum	35
VEGETABLES	Snap bean,frz,ckd,drnd,green 1 cup	35
VEGETABLES	Snap bean,frz,ckd,drnd,yellow 1 cup	35
VEGETABLES	Sweetpotatoes, cnned, vac pack1 piece	35
FRUITS	Tangerines, raw 1 tangrn	35
VEGETABLES	Dandelion greens, cooked, drnd1 cup	35
VEGETABLES	Squash, summer, cooked, draind1 cup	35
BREADS	Wheat, thin crackers 4 crackr	35
SWEETS	Whole-wheat wafers, crackers 2 crackr	35
SAUCES	Mayonnaise, imitation 1 tbsp	35
BREADS	Sandwich spread, pork, beef 1 tbsp	35
DAIRY	Butter, salted 1 pat	35
DAIRY	Butter, unsalted 1 pat	35
DAIRY	Margarine, regulr,hard,80% fat1 pat	35
FRUITS	Apricots, canned, juice pack 3 halves	40
VEGETABLES	Beet greens, cooked, drained 1 cup	40
BEVERAGES	Grapefruit, raw, pink 1/2 frut	40
BEVERAGES	Grapefruit, raw, white 1/2 frut	40
FRUITS	Grapes, european, raw, tokay 10 grape	40
FRUITS	Jams and preserves 1 pkt	40
FRUITS	Jellies 1 pkt	40
VEGETABLES	Onions, raw, sliced 1 cup	40
FRUITS	Pears, canned, juice pack 1 half	40
FRUITS	Raisins 1 packet	40
VEGETABLES	Spinach, cooked from raw, drnd1 cup	40
BEVERAGES	Tomato juice, canned w/o salt 1 cup	40
BEVERAGES	Tomato juice, canned with salt1 cup	40
VEGETABLES	Broccoli, raw 1 spear	40
SOUPS	Chicken noodle soup,dehyd,prpd1 pkt	40
VEGETABLES	Kale, cooked from frozen 1 cup	40
VEGETABLES	Kale, cooked from raw 1 cup	40
VEGETABLES	Mushrooms, cooked, drained 1 cup	40
SOUPS	Tomato veg soup, dehyd,prepred1 pkt	40
BREADS	Cheese crackers, sandwch,peant1 sandwh	40

CHART BY CALORIES

FOOD		Food Energy Calories
VEGETABLES	Broccoli, raw, cooked, drained1 cup	45
VEGETABLES	Carrots, raw, grated 1 cup	45
FRUITS	Honeydew melon, raw 1/10 mel	45
FRUITS	Kiwifruit, raw 1 kiwi	45
FRUITS	Pineapple, canned, heavy syrup1 slice	45
VEGETABLES	Sauerkraut, canned 1 cup	45
VEGETABLES	Snap bean,raw,ckd,drnd,green 1 cup	45
VEGETABLES	Snap bean,raw,ckd,drnd,yellow 1 cup	45
SWEETS	Sugar, white, granulated 1 tbsp	45
BEVERAGES	Vegetable juice cocktail, cnnd1 cup	45
VEGETABLES	Asparagus, ckd frm raw, dr,cut1 cup	45
FRUITS	Strawberries, raw 1 cup	45
POULTRY	Turkey loaf, breast meat w/o c2 slices	45
POULTRY	Turkey loaf, breast meat, w/ c2 slices	45
SPICES	Sesame seeds 1 tbsp	45
MEATS	Vienna sausage 1 sausag	45
DAIRY	Whipping cream, unwhiped,light1 tbsp	45
FRUITS	Apricots, raw 3 aprcot	50
VEGETABLES	Broccoli, frzn, cooked, draned1 cup	50
FRUITS	Jellies 1 tbsp	50
VEGETABLES	Pumpkin, cooked from raw 1 cup	50
VEGETABLES	Asparagus, ckd frm frz,drn,cut1 cup	50
VEGETABLES	Broccoli, raw, cooked, drained1 spear	50
FRUITS	Cherries, sweet, raw 10 chery	50
FRUITS	Lemon juice, canned 1 cup	50
FRUITS	Lime juice,canned 1 cup	50
BREADS	Saltines 4 crackr	50
VEGETABLES	Spinach, canned, drnd,w/ salt 1 cup	50
VEGETABLES	Spinach, canned, drnd,w/o salt1 cup	50
VEGETABLES	Tomatoes, canned, s+l, w/ salt1 cup	50
VEGETABLES	Tomatoes, canned, s+l,w/o salt1 cup	50
VEGETABLES	Turnip greens, cked frm frozen1 cup	50
FRUITS	Watermelon, raw, diced 1 cup	50
BREADS	Cheese crackers, plain 10 crack	50
MEATS	Pork, link, cooked 1 link	50
MEATS	Brown and serve sausage,brwnd 1 link	50
DAIRY	Margarine, imitation 40% fat 1 tbsp	50
DAIRY	Whipping cream, unwhiped,heavy1 tbsp	50
VEGETABLES	Artichokes, globe, cooked, drn1 artchk	55
VEGETABLES	Beets, canned, drained,no salt1 cup	55
VEGETABLES	Beets, canned, drained,w/ salt1 cup	55

CHART BY CALORIES

	FOOD	Food Energy Calories
VEGETABLES	Beets, cooked, drained, diced 1 cup	55
VEGETABLES	Carrots, cooked from frozen 1 cup	55
FRUITS	Jams and preserves 1 tbsp	55
VEGETABLES	Onions, raw, chopped 1 cup	55
FRUITS	Plums, canned, juice pack 3 plums	55
VEGETABLES	Spinach, cooked fr frzen, drnd1 cup	55
BEVERAGES	Lemon juice,frzn,single-strngh6 fl oz	55
BREADS	Rye wafers, whole-grain 2 wafers	55
BREADS	White bread, slice 22 per loaf1 slice	55
BREADS	White bread, toasted 22 per 1 slice	55
BREADS	Pancakes, buckwheat, from mix 1 pancak	55
NUTS	Popcorn, popped, veg oil,saltd1 cup	55
VEGETABLES	Corn, cooked frm frozn, white 1 ear	60
VEGETABLES	Corn, cooked frm frozn, yellow1 ear	60
FRUITS	Lemon juice, raw 1 cup	60
VEGETABLES	Onions, raw, cooked, drained 1 cup	60
FRUITS	Oranges, raw 1 orange	60
FRUITS	Peaches, canned, heavy syrup 1 half	60
FRUITS	Pears, canned, heavy syrup 1 half	60
VEGETABLES	Brussels sprouts, raw, cooked 1 cup	60
VEGETABLES	Collards, cooked from frozen 1 cup	60
SWEETS	Graham cracker, plain 2 crackr	60
FRUITS	Raspberries, raw 1 cup	60
SOUPS	Chicken rice soup, canned 1 cup	60
BREADS	Pancakes, plain, from mix 1 pancak	60
BREADS	Pancakes, plain, home recipe 1 pancak	60
DAIRY	Eggs, raw, yolk 1 yolk	60
SAUCES	Mayonnaise type salad dressing1 tbsp	60
SAUCES	1000 island, salad drsng,reglr1 tbsp	60
FRUITS	Apples, raw, peeled, sliced 1 cup	65
SWEETS	Honey 1 tbsp	65
FRUITS	Lime juice, raw 1 cup	65
FRUITS	Papayas, raw 1 cup	65
VEGETABLES	Peas, edible pod, cooked,drned1 cup	65
VEGETABLES	Brussels sprouts, frzn, cooked1 cup	65
FISH	Clams, raw 3 oz	65
BREADS	Cracked-wheat bread 1 slice	65
BREADS	Cracked-wheat bread, toasted 1 slice	65
BREADS	Mixed grain bread 1 slice	65
BREADS	Mixed grain bread, toasted 1 slice	65
FRUITS	Nectarines, raw 1 nectrn	65

CHART BY CALORIES

	FOOD		Food Energy Calories
BREADS	Oatmeal bread	1 slice	65
BREADS	Oatmeal bread, toasted	1 slice	65
BREADS	Pretzels, twisted, dutch	1 pretz	65
BREADS	Raisin bread	1 slice	65
BREADS	Raisin bread, toasted	1 slice	65
BREADS	Rye bread, light	1 slice	65
BREADS	Rye bread, light, toasted	1 slice	65
BREADS	Tortillas, corn	1 tortla	65
BREADS	Wheat bread	1 slice	65
BREADS	Wheat bread, toasted	1 slice	65
BREADS	White bread, slice 18 per loaf	1 slice	65
BREADS	White bread, toasted 18 per	1 slice	65
BREADS	Baking pwdr biscuits,refrgdogh	1 biscut	65
FRUITS	Apricot, canned, heavy syrup	3 halves	70
VEGETABLES	Carrots, cooked from raw	1 cup	70
MISCELLANEOUS	Gelatin dessert, prepared	1/2 cup	70
NUTS	Water chestnuts, canned	1 cup	70
CEREAL	All-bran cereal	1 oz	70
VEGETABLES	Lettuce, crisphead, raw, head	1 head	70
BREADS	Vienna bread	1 slice	70
SWEETS	Whole-wheat bread	1 slice	70
SWEETS	Whole-wheat bread, toasted	1 slice	70
SOUPS	Vegetarian soup, canned	1 cup	70
FISH	Fish sticks, frozen, reheated	1 stick	70
DAIRY	Cheddar cheese	1 cu in	70
SAUCES	Vinegar and oil salad dressing	1 tbsp	70
BEVERAGES	Limeade,concen,frozen,diluted	6 fl oz	75
FRUITS	Peaches, raw, sliced	1 cup	75
SAUCES	Tomato sauce, canned with salt	1 cup	75
VEGETABLES	Vegetables, mixed, canned	1 cup	75
BEVERAGES	Wine, table, red	3.5 f oz	75
FRUITS	Blackberries, raw	1 cup	75
SWEETS	Coca pwdr w/o nonfat dry milk	3/4 oz	75
FRUITS	Pineapple, raw, diced	1 cup	75
SOUPS	Chicken noodle soup, canned	1 cup	75
POULTRY	Chicken, roasted, drumstick	1.6 oz	75
MEATS	Pork, luncheon meat,ckd ham,ln	2 slices	75
POULTRY	Turkey ham, cured turkey thigh	2 slices	75
DAIRY	Eggs, cooked, hard-cooked	1 egg	75
DAIRY	Eggs, cooked, poached	1 egg	75
DAIRY	Eggs, raw, whole	1 egg	75

CHART BY CALORIES

FOOD		Food Energy Calories
DAIRY	Margarine, spread,hard,60% fat1 tbsp	75
DAIRY	Margarine, spread,soft,60% fat1 tbsp	75
FRUITS	Apples, raw, unpeeled,3 per lb1 apple	80
BREADS	Corn grits, cooked, instant 1 pkt	80
BEVERAGES	Lemonade,concen,frzen,diluted 6 fl oz	80
BEVERAGES	Wine, table, white 3.5 f oz	80
FRUITS	Blueberries, raw 1 cup	80
FISH	Flounder or sole, baked,w/ofat3 oz	80
BREADS	Pumpernickel bread 1 slice	80
BREADS	Pumpernickel bread, toasted 1 slice	80
VEGETABLES	Squash, winter, baked 1 cup	80
BREADS	White bread cubes 1 cup	80
SAUCES	Brown gravy from dry mix 1 cup	80
SOUPS	Clam chowder, manhattan, cannd1 cup	80
VEGETABLES	Seaweed, spirulina, dried 1 oz	80
SOUPS	Vegetable beef soup, canned 1 cup	80
SOUPS	Minestrone soup, canned 1 cup	80
DAIRY	Mozzarella chese,skim, lomoist1 oz	80
VEGETABLES	Onion rings, breaded,frzn,prpd2 rings	80
DAIRY	Mozzarella cheese, whole milk 1 oz	80
DAIRY	Pasterzd proces chese spred,am1 oz	80
SAUCES	Italian salad dressing,regular1 tbsp	80
BEVERAGES	Fruit punch drink, canned 6 fl oz	85
BREADS	Italian bread 1 slice	85
DAIRY	Milk, skim, no added milksolid1 cup	85
SWEETS	Molasses, cane, blackstrap 2 tbsp	85
FRUITS	Oranges, raw, sections 1 cup	85
SWEETS	Syrup, chocolate flavored thin2 tbsp	85
BEVERAGES	Tea,instant,prepard,sweetened 8 fl oz	85
VEGETABLES	Corn, cooked from raw, white 1 ear	85
VEGETABLES	Corn, cooked from raw, yellow 1 ear	85
DAIRY	Malted milk, chocolate, powder3/4 oz	85
FRUITS	Pears, raw, bosc 1 pear	85
VEGETABLES	Pumpkin, canned 1 cup	85
CEREAL	Raisin bran, post 1 oz	85
SAUCES	Chicken gravy from dry mix 1 cup	85
FISH	Clams, canned, drained 3 oz	85
DAIRY	Malted milk,natural, powder 3/4 oz	85
BREADS	Rolls, dinner, commercial 1 roll	85
SOUPS	Tomato soup w/ water, canned 1 cup	85
SOUPS	Beef noodle soup, canned 1 cup	85

CHART BY CALORIES

FOOD		Food Energy Calories
MEATS	Pork, cured, bacon,canadn,cked2 slice	85
DAIRY	Tofu 1 piece	85
MEATS	Salami, dry type 2 slices	85
SAUCES	French salad dressing, regular1 tbsp	85
CEREAL	Bran flakes, post 1 oz	90
FRUITS	Cherries, sour,red,cannd,water1 cup	90
SWEETS	Marshmallows 1 oz	90
BEVERAGES	Pineapple-grapefruit juicedrnk6 fl oz	90
CEREAL	Bran flakes, kellogg's 1 oz	90
DAIRY	Milk, skim, added milk solids 1 cup	90
CEREAL	Raisin bran, kellogg's 1 oz	90
POULTRY	Chicken roll, light 2 slices	90
FISH	Oysters, breaded, fried 1 oyster	90
DAIRY	Eggs, cooked, fried 1 egg	90
BEVERAGES	Beer, light 12 fl oz	95
POULTRY	Chicken chow mein, canned 1 cup	95
BEVERAGES	Gin,rum,vodka,whisky 80-proof 1.5 f oz	95
BEVERAGES	Grapefruit juice, canned,unswt1 cup	95
BEVERAGES	Grapefruit juice, raw 1 cup	95
BREADS	Boston brown bread,w/whtecrnm 1 slice	95
BREADS	Boston brown bread,w/yllwcrnml1 slice	95
FRUITS	Cantaloup, raw 1/2 meln	95
BREADS	Baking pwdr biscuits,from mix 1 biscut	95
SAUCES	Gravy and turkey, frozen 5 oz	95
SWEETS	Brownies w/ nuts,frm home recp1 browne	95
DAIRY	Pasterzd proces cheese, swiss 1 oz	95
DAIRY	Pasterzd proces chese food,amr1 oz	95
MEATS	Pork, luncheon meat,choppd ham2 slices	95
NUTS	Peanut butter 1 tbsp	95
DAIRY	Cream of wheat,ckd,mix n eat 1 pkt	100
BEVERAGES	Grape drink, canned 6 fl oz	100
BEVERAGES	Grapefrt jce,frzn,dltd,unswten1 cup	100
CEREAL	Grape-nuts cereal 1 oz	100
SWEETS	Gum drops 1 oz	100
CEREAL	Wheaties cereal 1 oz	100
SWEETS	Cocoa pwdr w/ nofat drmlk,prpd1 servng	100
SWEETS	Cocoa pwdr with nonfat drymilk1 oz	100
BREADS	French bread 1 slice	100
FRUITS	Pears, raw, bartlett 1 pear	100
CEREAL	Shredded wheat cereal 1 oz	100
FISH	Shrimp, canned, drained 3 oz	100

CHART BY CALORIES

FOOD			Food Energy Calories
CEREAL	Total cereal	1 oz	100
DAIRY	Buttermilk, fluid	1 cup	100
DAIRY	Milk, lofat, 1%, no addedsolid1 cup		100
SWEETS	Brownies w/ nuts,frstng,cmmrcl1 browne		100
BREADS	Baking pwdr biscuits,homerecpe1 biscut		100
DAIRY	Ice cream, vanlla, regulr 11% 3 fl oz		100
DAIRY	Eggs, cooked, scrambled/omelet1 egg		100
DAIRY	Blue cheese	1 oz	100
DAIRY	Provolone cheese	1 oz	100
DAIRY	Cream cheese	1 oz	100
DAIRY	Butter, salted	1 tbsp	100
DAIRY	Butter, unsalted	1 tbsp	100
DAIRY	Margarine, regulr,hard,80% fat1 tbsp		100
DAIRY	Margarine, regulr,soft,80% fat1 tbsp		100
SAUCES	Mayonnaise, regular	1 tbsp	100
FRUITS	Applesauce, canned,unsweetened1 cup		105
BEVERAGES	Gin,rum,vodka,whisky 86-proof 1.5 f oz		105
SWEETS	Jelly beans	1 oz	105
BEVERAGES	Orange + grapefruit juce,cannd1 cup		105
BEVERAGES	Orange juice, canned	1 cup	105
CEREAL	Super sugar crisp cereal	1 oz	105
SAUCES	Tomato puree, canned w/o salt 1 cup		105
SAUCES	Tomato puree, canned with salt1 cup		105
VEGETABLES	Vegetables, mixed, cked fr frz1 cup		105
FRUITS	Bananas	1 banana	105
CEREAL	Honey nut cheerios cereal	1 oz	105
CEREAL	Sugar smacks cereal	1 oz	105
DAIRY	Milk, lofat, 1%, added solids 1 cup		105
BREADS	Oatmeal,ckd,instnt,plain,fortf1 pkt		105
MEATS	Pork, cured, ham, rosted,lean 2.4 oz		105
SWEETS	Snack cakes,devils food,cremflsm cake		105
MEATS	Pork, luncheon meat,ckd ham,rg2 slices		105
BREADS	Potato chips	10 chips	105
DAIRY	Swiss cheese	1 oz	105
DAIRY	Muenster cheese	1 oz	105
DAIRY	Pasterzd proces cheese,americn1 oz		105
CEREAL	Corn flakes, kellogg's	1 oz	110
CEREAL	Corn flakes, toasties	1 oz	110
BEVERAGES	Gin,rum,vodka,whisky 90-proof 1.5 f oz		110
SWEETS	Hard candy	1 oz	110
BEVERAGES	Orange juice, raw	1 cup	110

CHART BY CALORIES

FOOD			Food Energy Calories
BEVERAGES	Orange juice,frzn,cncn,diluted1 cup		110
FRUITS	Peaches, canned, juice pack	1 cup	110
CEREAL	Product 19 cereal	1 oz	110
BREADS	Rice krispies cereal	1 oz	110
CEREAL	Special K cereal	1 oz	110
CEREAL	Sugar frosted flakes, kellogg	1 oz	110
CEREAL	Trix cereal	1 oz	110
CEREAL	Froot loops cereal	1 oz	110
CEREAL	Golden grahams cereal	1 oz	110
BREADS	Lucky charms cereal	1 oz	110
BEVERAGES	Orange juice, chilled	1 cup	110
CEREAL	Cheerios cereal	1 oz	110
VEGETABLES	Potatoes,french-frd,frzn,oven 10 strip		110
SWEETS	Pound cake, commercial	1 slice	110
BREADS	Danish pastry, plain, no nuts 1 oz		110
MEATS	Pork, cured, bacon, regul,cked3 slice		110
BEVERAGES	Apple juice, canned	1 cup	115
FRUITS	Fruit cocktail,cnnd,juice pack1 cup		115
BEVERAGES	Grapefruit juice, canned,swtnd1 cup		115
VEGETABLES	Jerusalem-artichoke, raw	1 cup	115
PASTA	Macaroni, cooked, tender,cold 1 cup		115
VEGETABLES	Potatoes, boiled, peeled befor1 potato		115
FRUITS	Prunes, dried	5 large	115
VEGETABLES	Sweetpotatoes, baked, peeled 1 potato		115
VEGETABLES	Peas, green,cnnd,drnd, w/ salt1 cup		115
VEGETABLES	Peas, green,cnnd,drnd,w/o salt1 cup		115
BREADS	Rolls, frankfurter + hamburger1 roll		115
SWEETS	Caramels, plain or chocolate	1 oz	115
SWEETS	Fudge, chocolate, plain	1 oz	115
SOUPS	Cr of chicken soup w/ h20,cnnd1 cup		115
DAIRY	Camembert cheese	1 wedge	115
DAIRY	Cheddar cheese	1 oz	115
POULTRY	Chicken frankfurter	1 frank	115
SAUCES	Fats, cooking/vegetbl shorteng1 tbsp		115
DAIRY	Lard	1 tbsp	115
FRUITS	Apricots, canned, juice pack	1 cup	120
BREADS	Cornmeal,degermed,enriched,cook1 cup		120
FRUITS	Plums, canned, heavy syrup	3 plums	120
VEGETABLES	Potatoes, boiled, peeled after1 potato		120
FRUITS	Pears, raw, d'anjou	1 pear	120
BREADS	White bread crumbs, soft	1 cup	120

CHART BY CALORIES

	FOOD	Food Energy Calories
CEREAL	Cap'n crunch cereal 1 oz	120
BREADS	Rolls, dinner, home recipe 1 roll	120
SWEETS	Devil's food cake,chocfrst,fmx1 cupcak	120
DAIRY	Milk, lofat, 2%, no addedsolid1 cup	120
SWEETS	Pound cake, from home recipe 1 slice	120
FISH	Salmon, canned, pink, w/ bones3 oz	120
FISH	Flounder or sole, baked, buttr3 oz	120
FISH	Flounder or sole, baked,margrn3 oz	120
SAUCES	Mushroom gravy, canned 1 cup	120
POULTRY	Chicken, fried, flour, drmstck1.7 oz	120
SWEETS	Table syrup (corn and maple) 2 tbsp	122
SWEETS	Angelfood cake, from mix 1 piece	125
BEVERAGES	Ginger ale 12 fl oz	125
BEVERAGES	Grapejce,frzn,dilutd,swtnd,w/c1 cup	125
VEGETABLES	Parsnips, cooked, drained 1 cup	125
FRUITS	Pears, canned, juice pack 1 cup	125
VEGETABLES	Peas,grn, frozen cooked,draned1 cup	125
FRUITS	Tangerine juice, canned,swtned1 cup	125
DAIRY	Yogurt, w/ nonfat milk 8 oz	125
FRUITS	Apples, raw, unpeeled,2 per lb1 apple	125
DAIRY	Cottage cheese,uncreamed 1 cup	125
SAUCES	Beef gravy, canned 1 cup	125
DAIRY	Milk, lofat, 2%, added solids 1 cup	125
CEREAL	Nature valley granola cereal 1 oz	125
SWEETS	Syrup, chocolate flvred, fudge2 tbsp	125
BREADS	Bran muffins, home recipe 1 muffin	125
SAUCES	Corn oil 1 tbsp	125
SAUCES	Olive oil 1 tbsp	125
SAUCES	Peanut oil 1 tbsp	125
OILS	Safflower oil 1 tbsp	125
SAUCES	Soybean oil, hydrogenated 1 tbsp	125
SAUCES	Soybean-cottonseed oil, hydrgn1 tbsp	125
OILS	Sunflower oil 1 tbsp	125
POULTRY	Turkey roast, frzn,lght+drk,ck3 oz	130
MEATS	Lamb, rib, roasted, lean only 2 oz	130
SOUPS	Cr of mushrom soup w/ h2o,cnnd1 cup	130
DAIRY	Parmesan cheese, grated 1 oz	130
VEGETABLES	Corn, cooked frm frozn, white 1 cup	135
VEGETABLES	Corn, cooked frm frozn, yellow1 cup	135
VEGETABLES	Mangos, raw 1 mango	135
NUTS	Popcorn, sugar syrup coated 1 cup	135

CHART BY CALORIES

FOOD		Food Energy Calories
FISH	Tuna, cannd, drnd,watr, white 3 oz	135
FISH	Crabmeat, canned 1 cup	135
POULTRY	Turkey, roasted, light meat 2 pieces	135
MEATS	Beef roast, eye o rnd, lean 2.6 oz	135
SWEETS	Blueberry muffins, home recipe1 muffin	135
CEREAL	100% natural cereal 1 oz	135
MEATS	Lamb,chops,arm,braised,lean 1.7 oz	135
FRUITS	Apricot nectar, no added vit c1 cup	140
DAIRY	Crm wheat,ckd, quick, no salt 1 cup	140
DAIRY	Crm wheat,ckd,quick, w/ salt 1 cup	140
DAIRY	Crm wheat,ckd,reg,inst,no salt1 cup	140
DAIRY	Crm wheat,ckd,reg,inst,w/salt 1 cup	140
BEVERAGES	Pineapple juice, canned,unswtn1 cup	140
BEVERAGES	Wine, dessert 3.5 f oz	140
FRUITS	Bananas, sliced 1 cup	140
BREADS	English muffins, plain 1 muffin	140
BREADS	English muffins, plain, toastd1 muffin	140
POULTRY	Chicken, roasted, breast 3.0 oz	140
BREADS	Bran muffins, from commerl mix1 muffin	140
SWEETS	Blueberry muffins,from com mix1 muffin	140
FISH	Salmon, baked, red 3 oz	140
FISH	Halibut, broiled, butter,lemju3 oz	140
MEATS	Lamb,chops,loin,broil,lean 2.3 oz	140
MEATS	Lamb,leg,roasted, lean only 2.6 oz	140
SWEETS	Milk chocolate candy,w/ rice c1 oz	140
MEATS	Pork, cured, ham, canned,roast3 oz	140
DAIRY	Yogurt, w/ whole milk 8 oz	140
MEATS	Pork, luncheon meat,canned 2 slices	140
BREADS	Corn grits,ckd,reg,whte,nosalt1 cup	145
BREADS	Corn grits,ckd,reg,whte,w/salt1 cup	145
BREADS	Corn grits,ckd,reg,yllw,nosalt1 cup	145
BREADS	Corn grits,ckd,reg,yllw,w/salt1 cup	145
BEVERAGES	Cranberry juice cocktal w/vitc1 cup	145
FRUITS	Plums, canned, juice pack 1 cup	145
VEGETABLES	Potatoes, baked flesh only 1 potato	145
BREADS	Oatmeal,ckd,rg,qck,inst,w/osal1 cup	145
BREADS	Oatmeal,ckd,rg,qck,inst,w/salt1 cup	145
VEGETABLES	Sweetpotatoes, candied 1 piece	145
MEATS	Beef, dried, chipped 2.5 oz	145
DAIRY	Pudding, tapioca, from mix 1/2 cup	145
DAIRY	Pudding, vnlla,cooked from mix1/2 cup	145

CHART BY CALORIES

FOOD		Food Energy Calories
POULTRY	Turkey, roasted, light + dark 3 pieces	145
DAIRY	Yogurt, w/ lofat milk, plain 8 oz	145
BREADS	Corn muffins, from commerl mix1 muffin	145
SWEETS	Shortbread cookie, home recipe2 cookie	145
SWEETS	Milk chocolate candy, plain 1 oz	145
MEATS	Salami, cooked type 2 slices	145
MEATS	Frankfurter, cooked 1 frank	145
SWEETS	Chocolate, bitter ot baking 1 oz	145
BEVERAGES	Beer, regular 12 fl oz	150
BEVERAGES	Grapefruit, canned, syrup pack1 cup	150
FRUITS	Pineapple, canned, juice pack 1 cup	150
DAIRY	Pudding, choc, cooked from mix1/2 cup	150
DAIRY	Pudding, vnlla,instant frm mix1/2 cup	150
MEATS	Beef heart, braised 3 oz	150
MEATS	Beef steak,sirloin,broil,lean 2.5 oz	150
DAIRY	Milk, whole, 3.3% fat 1 cup	150
FISH	Salmon, smoked 3 oz	150
MEATS	Beef roast, rib, lean only 2.2 oz	150
DAIRY	Imitatn whipd toping,pwdrd,prp1 cup	150
SWEETS	Milk chocolate candy,w/ almond1 oz	150
SWEETS	Sweet (dark) chocolate 1 oz	150
FRUITS	Apples, dried, sulfured 10 rings	155
BEVERAGES	Grape juice, canned 1 cup	155
BEVERAGES	Lemon-lime soda 12 fl oz	155
FRUITS	Tangerines, canned, light syrp1 cup	155
PASTA	Macaroni, cooked, tender, hot 1 cup	155
PASTA	Spaghetti, cooked, tender 1 cup	155
BREADS	Rolls, hard 1 roll	155
FRUITS	Watermelon, raw 1 piece	155
DAIRY	Pudding, choc, instant, fr mix1/2 cup	155
DAIRY	Pudding, rice, from mix 1/2 cup	155
SWEETS	Snack cakes,sponge creme fllngsm cake	155
BREADS	French toast, home recipe 1 slice	155
BREADS	Corn chips 1 oz	155
SWEETS	Milk chocolate candy,w/ penuts1 oz	155
VEGETABLES	Pumpkin and squash kernels 1 oz	155
DAIRY	Whipped topping, pressurized 1 cup	155
BEVERAGES	Cola, regular 12 fl oz	160
BEVERAGES	Pepper-type soda 12 fl oz	160
VEGETABLES	Sweetpotatoes, boiled w/o peel1 potato	160
VEGETABLES	Potatoes, mashed,recpe,w/ milk1 cup	160

CHART BY CALORIES

FOOD		Food Energy Calories
BREADS	Oatmeal,ckd,instnt,flvrd,fortf1 pkt	160
BEVERAGES	Chocolate milk, lowfat 1% 1 cup	160
FISH	Oysters, raw 1 cup	160
DAIRY	Pudding, tapioca, canned 5 oz	160
SOUPS	Tomato soup with milk, canned 1 cup	160
POULTRY	Turkey, roasted, dark meat 4 pieces	160
MEATS	Pork fresh ham, roastd, lean 2.5 oz	160
VEGETABLES	Potatoes,french-frd,frzn,fried10 strip	160
NUTS	Sunflower seeds 1 oz	160
SWEETS	Coconut, raw, piece 1 piece	160
NUTS	Pine nuts 1 oz	160
BEVERAGES	Root beer 12 fl oz	165
VEGETABLES	Corn,cnnd,whl krnl,whte,no sal1 cup	165
VEGETABLES	Corn,cnnd,whl krnl,whte,w/salt1 cup	165
VEGETABLES	Corn,cnnd,whl krnl,yllw,no sal1 cup	165
VEGETABLES	Corn,cnnd,whl krnl,yllw,w/salt1 cup	165
BREADS	Pita bread 1 pita	165
SOUPS	Pea, green, soup, canned 1 cup	165
SOUPS	Clam chowder, new eng, w/ milk1 cup	165
SWEETS	Fruitcake,dark, from homerecip1 piece	165
FISH	Tuna, cannd, drnd,oil,chk,lght3 oz	165
MEATS	Pork chop, loin, broil, lean 2.5 oz	165
MEATS	Pork shoulder, braisd, lean 2.4 oz	165
NUTS	Cashew nuts, dry roastd,salted1 oz	165
NUTS	Cashew nuts, dry roastd,unsalt1 oz	165
NUTS	Cashew nuts, oil roastd,salted1 oz	165
NUTS	Cashew nuts, oil roastd,unsalt1 oz	165
NUTS	Peanuts, oil roasted, salted 1 oz	165
NUTS	Peanuts, oil roasted, unsalted1 oz	165
NUTS	Pistachio nuts 1 oz	165
NUTS	Almonds, whole 1 oz	165
SWEETS	Popsicle 1 popcle	170
VEGETABLES	Lima beans,thick seed,frzn,ckd1 cup	170
VEGETABLES	Bean with bacon soup, canned 1 cup	170
MEATS	Beef, ckd,chuck blade,leanonly2.2 oz	170
NUTS	Mixed nuts w/ peants,dry,saltd1 oz	170
NUTS	Mixed nuts w/ peants,dry,unslt1 oz	170
NUTS	Walnuts, black, chopped 1 oz	170
SWEETS	Gingerbread cake, from mix 1 piece	175
MEATS	Beef, ckd,bttm round,lean only2.8 oz	175
FISH	Haddock, breaded, fried 3 oz	175

CHART BY CALORIES

	FOOD		Food Energy Calories
FISH	Sardines, atlntc,cnned,oil,drn3 oz		175
FISH	Trout, broiled, w/ buttr,lemju3 oz		175
MEATS	Pork fresh rib, roastd, lean 2.5 oz		175
NUTS	Mixed nuts w/ peants,oil,saltd1 oz		175
NUTS	Mixed nuts w/ peants,oil,unslt1 oz		175
BEVERAGES	Grape soda	12 fl oz	180
VEGETABLES	Orange soda	12 fl oz	180
FRUITS	Plantains, cooked	1 cup	180
FRUITS	Prune juice, canned	1 cup	180
RICE	Rice, white, instant, cooked 1 cup		180
VEGETABLES	Blackeye peas, immatr,raw,cked1 cup		180
BEVERAGES	Chocolate milk, lowfat 2%	1 cup	180
SWEETS	Chocolate chip cookies,commrcl4 cookie		180
MEATS	Pork chop, loin,panfry, lean 2.4 oz		180
POULTRY	Turkey patties, brd,battd,frid1 patty		180
MEATS	Bologna	2 slices	180
NUTS	Filberts, (hazelnuts) chopped 1 oz		180
NUTS	Walnuts, english, pieces	1 oz	180
FRUITS	Blueberries, frozen, sweetened1 cup		185
FRUITS	Fruit cocktail,cnnd,heavysyrup1 cup		185
RICE	Rice, white, parboiled, cooked1 cup		185
VEGETABLES	Corn, cnnd,crm stl,whit,no sal1 cup		185
VEGETABLES	Corn, cnnd,crm stl,whit,w/salt1 cup		185
VEGETABLES	Corn, cnnd,crm stl,yllw,no sal1 cup		185
VEGETABLES	Corn, cnnd,crm stl,yllw,w/salt1 cup		185
DAIRY	Ice milk, vanilla, 4% fat	1 cup	185
MEATS	Beef liver, fried	3 oz	185
SWEETS	Vanilla wafers	10 cooke	185
MEATS	Veal cutlet, med fat,brsd,brld3 oz		185
MEATS	Beef, canned, corned	3 oz	185
SWEETS	Chocolate chip cookies,hme rcp4 cookie		185
FISH	Ocean perch, breaded, fried 1 fillet		185
DAIRY	Imitatn whipd toping,pressrzd 1 cup		185
NUTS	Brazil nuts	1 oz	185
FRUITS	Peaches, canned, heavy syrup 1 cup		190
FRUITS	Pears, canned, heavy syrup	1 cup	190
VEGETABLES	Black-eyed peas, dry, cooked 1 cup		190
VEGETABLES	Lima beans,baby, frzn,cked,drn1 cup		190
PASTA	Macaroni, cooked, firm	1 cup	190
PASTA	Spaghetti, cooked, firm	1 cup	190
PASTA	Spaghetti, tom sauce chees,cnd1 cup		190

CHART BY CALORIES

FOOD		Food Energy Calories
SOUPS	Cr of chicken soup w/ mlk,cnnd1 cup	190
FISH	Herring, pickled 3 oz	190
SAUCES	Chicken gravy, canned 1 cup	190
NUTS	Pecans, halves 1 oz	190
FRUITS	Applesauce, canned, sweetened 1 cup	195
SWEETS	Sandwich type cookie 4 cookie	195
FISH	Scallops, breaded, frzn,reheat6 scalop	195
POULTRY	Chicken, fried, batter,drmstck2.5 oz	195
BREADS	Taco 1 taco	195
FRUITS	Pineapple, canned, heavy syrup1 cup	200
BEVERAGES	Evaporated milk, skim, canned 1 cup	200
FRUITS	Peaches, dried,cooked,unswetnd1 cup	200
BREADS	Bagels, egg 1 bagel	200
BREADS	Bagels, plain 1 bagel	200
PASTA	Noodles, egg, cooked 1 cup	200
FISH	Shrimp, french fried 3 oz	200
DAIRY	Cottage cheese,lowfat 2% 1 cup	205
BREADS	Waffles, from mix 1 waffle	205
DAIRY	Pudding, chocolate,canned 5 oz	205
MEATS	Beef roast, eye o rnd,lean+fat3 oz	205
MEATS	Lamb,leg,roasted, lean+ fat 3 oz	205
SOUPS	Cr of mushrom soup w/ mlk,cnnd1 cup	205
MEATS	Pork, cured, ham, rosted,ln+ft3 oz	205
MEATS	Braunschweiger 2 slices	205
NUTS	Macadamia nuts, oilrstd,salted1 oz	205
NUTS	Macadamia nuts, oilrstd,unsalt1 oz	205
FRUITS	Apricots, dried, cooked,unswtn1 cup	210
MISCELLANEOUS	Great northn beans,dry,ckd,drn1 cup	210
SWEETS	Fig bars 4 cookie	210
BREADS	Toaster pastries 1 pastry	210
BEVERAGES	Chocolate milk, regular 1 cup	210
VEGETABLES	Potatoes, scalloped, home recp1 cup	210
SWEETS	Doughnuts, cake type, plain 1 donut	210
FRUITS	Apricot, canned, heavy syrup 1 cup	215
VEGETABLES	Lentils, dry, cooked 1 cup	215
DAIRY	Cottage cheese,cremd,smll curd1 cup	215
VEGETABLES	Potatoes, baked with skin 1 potato	220
FRUITS	Plantains, raw 1 plantn	220
SAUCES	Tomato paste, canned w/o salt 1 cup	220
SAUCES	Tomato paste, canned with salt1 cup	220
POULTRY	Chicken, fried, flour, breast 3.5 oz	220

CHART BY CALORIES

	FOOD	Food Energy Calories
DAIRY	Pudding, vanilla, canned 5 oz	220
MEATS	Beef and vegetable stew,hm rcp1 cup	220
PASTA	Noodles, chow mein, canned 1 cup	220
BREADS	Danish pastry, plain, no nuts 1 pastry	220
MEATS	Beef, ckd,bttm round,lean+ fat3 oz	220
MEATS	Lamb,chops,arm,braised,lean+ft2.2 oz	220
VEGETABLES	Spinach souffle 1 cup	220
FRUITS	Prunes, dried, cooked,unswtned1 cup	225
RICE	Rice, white, cooked 1 cup	225
VEGETABLES	Black beans, dry, cooked,drand1 cup	225
VEGETABLES	Blackeye peas,immtr,frzn,cked 1 cup	225
VEGETABLES	Pea beans, dry, cooked,drained1 cup	225
DAIRY	Ice milk, vanilla,softserv 3% 1 cup	225
SWEETS	Coca pwdr w/o nofat drymlk,prd1 servng	225
VEGETABLES	Potatoes, mashed,recpe,mlk+mar1 cup	225
SWEETS	Chocolate chip cookies,refrig 4 cookie	225
FRUITS	Blueberries, frozen, sweetened10 oz	230
NUTS	Dates 10 dates	230
FRUITS	Plums, canned, heavy syrup 1 cup	230
VEGETABLES	Peas, split, dry, cooked 1 cup	230
VEGETABLES	Red kidney beans, dry, canned 1 cup	230
RICE	Rice, brown, cooked 1 cup	230
DAIRY	Yogurt, w/ lofat milk,fruitflv8 oz	230
BREADS	Coffeecake, crumb, from mix 1 piece	230
PASTA	Macaroni and cheese, canned 1 cup	230
VEGETABLES	Potatoes, au gratin, from mix 1 cup	230
VEGETABLES	Potatoes, scalloped, from mix 1 cup	230
MEATS	Veal rib, med fat, roasted 3 oz	230
MEATS	Ground beef, broiled, lean 3 oz	230
FRUITS	Peaches, frozen,swetned,w/vitc1 cup	235
SWEETS	Devil's food cake,chocfrst,fmx1 piece	235
SWEETS	Yellow cake w/ choc frst,frmix1 piece	235
DAIRY	Malted milk,chocolate, pwdrppd1 servng	235
DAIRY	Cottage cheese,cremd,lrge curd1 cup	235
DAIRY	Malted milk,natural, pwdr pprd1 servng	235
SAUCES	Soybeans, dry, cooked, drained1 cup	235
POULTRY	Chicken, canned, boneless 5 oz	235
BREADS	Croissants 1 crosst	235
VEGETABLES	Potatoes, mashed,frm dehydrted1 cup	235
SWEETS	Sugar cookie, from refrig dogh4 cookie	235
BREADS	Danish pastry, fruit 1 pastry	235

CHART BY CALORIES

	FOOD	Food Energy Calories
SWEETS	Doughnuts, yeast-leavend,glzed1 donut	235
BREADS	Enchilada 1 enchld	235
MEATS	Lamb,chops,loin,broil,lean+fat2.8 oz	235
BREADS	Pretzels, twisted, thin 10 pretz	240
POULTRY	Turkey, roasted, light + dark 1 cup	240
SWEETS	White sauce w/ milk from mix 1 cup	240
MEATS	Beef steak,sirloin,broil,ln+ft3 oz	240
DAIRY	Imitation whipped topping,frzn1 cup	240
SAUCES	Hollandaise sce, w/ h2o,frm mx1 cup	240
DAIRY	Nonfat dry milk, instantized 1 cup	245
FRUITS	Strawberries, frozen, sweetend1 cup	245
BREADS	Oatmeal w/ raisins cookies 4 cookie	245
MEATS	Hamburger, regular 1 sandwh	245
SWEETS	Yellowcake w/ chocfrstng,comml1 piece	245
BREADS	Waffles, from home recipe 1 waffle	245
NUTS	Peanut butter cookie,home recp4 cookie	245
MEATS	Ground beef, broiled, regular 3 oz	245
POULTRY	Chicken, stewed, light + dark 1 cup	250
SWEETS	Fried pie, cherry 1 pie	250
MEATS	Pork fresh ham, roastd,lean+ft3 oz	250
MISCELLANEOUS	Carob flour 1 cup	255
FRUITS	Raspberries, frozen, sweetened1 cup	255
POULTRY	Chicken chow mein, home recipe1 cup	255
SWEETS	Fried pie, apple 1 pie	255
VEGETABLES	Lima beans, dry, cooked,draned1 cup	260
VEGETABLES	Sweetpotatoes, canned, mashed 1 cup	260
PASTA	Spaghetti, tom sauce chee,hmrp1 cup	260
SWEETS	White cake w/ wht frstng,comml1 piece	260
PASTA	Spaghetti,meatballs,tomsac,cnd1 cup	260
FRUITS	Peaches, frozen,swetned,w/vitc10 oz	265
VEGETABLES	Pinto beans,dry,cooked,drained1 cup	265
VEGETABLES	Chickpeas, cooked, drained 1 cup	270
SWEETS	Sherbet, 2% fat 1 cup	270
DAIRY	Ice cream, vanlla, regulr 11% 1 cup	270
MEATS	Pork fresh rib, roastd,lean+ft3 oz	270
FRUITS	Strawberries, frozen, sweetend10 oz	275
MEATS	Pork chop, loin, broil, len+ft3.1 oz	275
FRUITS	Rhubarb, cooked, added sugar 1 cup	280
DAIRY	Cottage cheese,cremd,w/fruit 1 cup	280
SWEETS	Cheesecake 1 piece	280
SWEETS	Coconut, raw, shredded 1 cup	285

CHART BY CALORIES

	FOOD		Food Energy Calories
SAUCES	Catsup	1 cup	290
BREADS	Pizza, cheese	1 slice	290
FRUITS	Raspberries, frozen, sweetened	10 oz	295
VEGETABLES	Refried beans, canned	1 cup	295
MEATS	Pork shoulder, braisd,lean+fat	3 oz	295
BEVERAGES	Grapefrt jce,frzn,cncn,unswten	6 fl oz	300
MEATS	Cheeseburger, regular	1 sandwh	300
MEATS	Chop suey w/ beef + pork,hmrcp	1 cup	300
SWEETS	Custard, baked	1 cup	305
DAIRY	Cheese sauce w/ milk, frm mix	1 cup	305
VEGETABLES	Avocados, california	1 avocdo	305
FRUITS	Apricots, dried, uncooked	1 cup	310
VEGETABLES	Beans,dry,canned,w/pork+tomsce	1 cup	310
DAIRY	Shakes, thick, vanilla	10 oz	315
SWEETS	Sheetcake,w/o frstng,homerecip	1 piece	315
MEATS	Beef roast, rib, lean + fat	3 oz	315
MEATS	Lamb, rib, roasted, lean + fat	3 oz	315
BEVERAGES	Half and half, cream	1 cup	315
SWEETS	Pumpkin pie	1 piece	320
DAIRY	Nonfat dry milk, instantized	1 envlpe	325
VEGETABLES	Potatoes, au gratin, home recp	1 cup	325
MEATS	Beef, ckd,chuck blade,lean+fat	3 oz	325
PASTA	Spaghetti,meatballs,tomsa,hmrp	1 cup	330
SWEETS	Custard pie	1 piece	330
DAIRY	Shakes, thick, chocolate	10 oz	335
MEATS	Pork chop, loin,panfry,lean+ft	3.1 oz	335
BEVERAGES	Orange juice,frozen concentrte	6 fl oz	340
MISCELLANEOUS	Buckwheat flour, light, sifted	1 cup	340
VEGETABLES	Chili con carne w/ beans, cnnd	1 cup	340
VEGETABLES	Potatoes, hashed brown,fr frzn	1 cup	340
BEVERAGES	Eggnog	1 cup	340
BEVERAGES	Evaporated milk, whole, canned	1 cup	340
DAIRY	Ricotta cheese, part skim milk	1 cup	340
VEGETABLES	Avocados, florida	1 avocdo	340
MEATS	Roast beef sandwich	1 sandwh	345
MISCELLANEOUS	Cake or pastry flour, sifted	1 cup	350
NUTS	Chestnuts, european, roasted	1 cup	350
DAIRY	Ice cream, vanlla, rich 16% ft	1 cup	350
SWEETS	Lemon meringue pie	1 piece	355
BREADS	Eng muffin, egg, cheese, bacon	1 sandwh	360
VEGETABLES	Potato salad made w/ mayonnais	1 cup	360

CHART BY CALORIES

FOOD		Food Energy Calories
VEGETABLES	Beans,dry,canned,w/frankfurter1 cup	365
POULTRY	Chicken and noodles, home recp1 cup	365
POULTRY	Chicken, fried, batter, breast4.9 oz	365
FISH	Tuna salad 1 cup	375
DAIRY	Ice cream, vanlla, soft serve 1 cup	375
FRUITS	Peaches, dried 1 cup	380
SWEETS	Blueberry pie 1 piece	380
SWEETS	Sugar, powdered, sifted 1 cup	385
BEVERAGES	Grapejce,frzn,concen,swtnd,w/c6 fl oz	385
VEGETABLES	Beans,dry,canned,w/pork+swtsce1 cup	385
SWEETS	Carrot cake,cremchese frst,rec1 piece	385
BREADS	Breadcrumbs, dry, grated 1 cup	390
SWEETS	White sauce, medium, home recp1 cup	395
SWEETS	Whole-wheat flour,hrd wht,stir1 cup	400
BREADS	Rolls, hoagie or submarine 1 roll	400
SWEETS	Peach pie 1 piece	405
SWEETS	Apple pie 1 piece	405
BEVERAGES	Limeade,concentrate,frzn,undil6 fl oz	410
SWEETS	Cherry pie 1 piece	410
DAIRY	Imitatn sour dressing 1 cup	415
FRUITS	Cranberry sauce, canned,swtnd 1 cup	420
BREADS	Wheat flour, all-purpose,siftd1 cup	420
FISH	Fish sandwich, reg, w/ cheese 1 sandwh	420
BREADS	Bread stuffing,from mx,moist 1 cup	420
BEVERAGES	Lemonade,concentrate,frz,undil6 fl oz	425
PASTA	Macaroni and cheese, home rcpe1 cup	430
DAIRY	Ricotta cheese, whole milk 1 cup	430
FRUITS	Raisins 1 cup	435
BREADS	Cornmeal,whole-grnd,unbolt,dry1 cup	435
BREADS	Self-rising flour, unsifted 1 cup	440
BREADS	Cornmeal,bolted,dry form 1 cup	440
SWEETS	Sheetcake,w/ whfrstng,homercip1 piece	445
MEATS	Hamburger, 4oz patty 1 sandwh	445
POULTRY	Duck, roasted, flesh only 1/2 duck	445
BREADS	Wheat flour, all-purpose,unsif1 cup	455
SWEETS	Creme pie 1 piece	455
DAIRY	Parmesan cheese, grated 1 cup	455
DAIRY	Chedddar cheese, shredded 1 cup	455
DAIRY	Buttermilk, dried 1 cup	465
FISH	Fish sandwich, lge, w/o cheese1 sandwh	470
SWEETS	Coconut, dried, sweetnd,shredd1 cup	470

CHART BY CALORIES

FOOD		Food Energy Calories
POULTRY	Chicken a la king, home recipe1 cup	470
DAIRY	Light, coffee or table cream 1 cup	470
FRUITS	Figs, dried 10 figs	475
NUTS	Dates, chopped 1 cup	490
DAIRY	Sour cream 1 cup	495
BREADS	Cornmeal,degermed,enriched,dry1 cup	500
BREADS	Bread stuffing,from mx,drytype1 cup	500
MEATS	Beef potpie, home recipe 1 piece	515
MEATS	Cheeseburger, 4oz patty 1 sandwh	525
POULTRY	Chicken potpie, home recipe 1 piece	545
SWEETS	Pecan pie 1 piece	575
PASTA	Bulgur, uncooked 1 cup	600
DAIRY	Quiche lorraine 1 slice	600
DAIRY	Margarine, spread,hard,60% fat1/2 cup	610
RICE	Rice, white, raw 1 cup	670
RICE	Rice, white, parboiled, raw 1 cup	685
VEGETABLES	Barley, pearled,light, uncookd1 cup	700
DAIRY	Whipping cream, unwhiped,light1 cup	700
NUTS	Pecans, halves 1 cup	720
NUTS	Filberts, (hazelnuts) chopped 1 cup	725
NUTS	Cashew nuts, oil roastd,salted1 cup	750
NUTS	Cashew nuts, oil roastd,unsalt1 cup	750
NUTS	Walnuts, black, chopped 1 cup	760
SWEETS	Sugar, white, granulated 1 cup	770
NUTS	Walnuts, english, pieces 1 cup	770
NUTS	Cashew nuts, dry roastd,unsalt1 cup	785
NUTS	Cashew nuts, dry roasted,saltd1 cup	785
DAIRY	Margarine, imitation 40% fat 8 oz	785
NUTS	Almonds, slivered 1 cup	795
DAIRY	Margarine, regulr,hard,80% fat1/2 cup	810
DAIRY	Butter, salted 1/2 cup	810
DAIRY	Butter, unsalted 1/2 cup	810
SWEETS	Sugar, brown, pressed down 1 cup	820
DAIRY	Whipping cream, unwhiped,heavy1 cup	820
NUTS	Peanuts, oil roasted, salted 1 cup	840
NUTS	Peanuts, oil roasted, unsalted1 cup	840
SWEETS	Semisweet chocolate 1 cup	860
BREADS	Piecrust,from home recipe 1 shell	900
NUTS	Macadamia nuts, oilrstd,salted1 cup	960
NUTS	Macadamia nuts, oilrstd,unsalt1 cup	960
SWEETS	Sweetened condensed milk cnnd 1 cup	980

CHART BY CALORIES

FOOD			Food Energy Calories
SWEETS	Honey	1 cup	1030
SWEETS	Whole-wheat bread	1 loaf	1110
BREADS	Oatmeal bread	1 loaf	1145
BREADS	Pumpernickel bread	1 loaf	1160
BREADS	Wheat bread	1 loaf	1160
BREADS	Mixed grain bread	1 loaf	1165
BREADS	Cracked-wheat bread	1 loaf	1190
BREADS	Rye bread, light	1 loaf	1190
BREADS	White bread	1 loaf	1210
DAIRY	Margarine, spread,soft,60% fat	8 oz	1225
BREADS	Italian bread	1 loaf	1255
BREADS	Raisin bread	1 loaf	1260
BREADS	French or vienna bread	1 loaf	1270
BREADS	Danish pastry, plain, no nuts	1 ring	1305
BREADS	Coffeecake, crumb, from mix	1 cake	1385
DAIRY	Ice milk, vanilla, 4% fat	1/2 gal	1470
BREADS	Piecrust, from mix	2 crust	1485
SWEETS	Angelfood cake, from mix	1 cake	1510
SWEETS	Shortbread cookie, commercial	4 cookie	1556
SWEETS	Gingerbread cake, from mix	1 cake	1575
DAIRY	Margarine, regulr,soft,80% fat	8 oz	1625
SAUCES	Fats, cooking/vegetbl shorteng	1 cup	1810
DAIRY	Lard	1 cup	1850
SAUCES	Olive oil	1 cup	1910
SAUCES	Peanut oil	1 cup	1910
SWEETS	Pumpkin pie	1 pie	1920
SAUCES	Corn oil	1 cup	1925
OILS	Safflower oil	1 cup	1925
SAUCES	Soybean oil, hydrogenated	1 cup	1925
SAUCES	Soybean-cottonseed oil, hydrgn	1 cup	1925
OILS	Sunflower oil	1 cup	1925
SWEETS	Pound cake, commercial	1 loaf	1935
SWEETS	Custard pie	1 pie	1985
SWEETS	Pound cake, from home recipe	1 loaf	2025
SWEETS	Lemon meringue pie	1 pie	2140
DAIRY	Ice cream, vanlla, regulr 11%	1/2 galn	2155
SWEETS	Sherbet, 2% fat	1/2 gal	2160
SWEETS	Blueberry pie	1 pie	2285
SWEETS	Peach pie	1 pie	2410
SWEETS	Apple pie	1 pie	2420
SWEETS	Cherry pie	1 pie	2465

CHART BY CALORIES

	FOOD		Food Energy Calories
SWEETS	Creme pie	1 pie	2710
DAIRY	Ice cream, vanlla, rich 16% ft1/2 gal		2805
SWEETS	Sheetcake w/o frstng,homerecip1 cake		2830
SWEETS	Cheesecake	1 cake	3350
SWEETS	Pecan pie	1 pie	3450
SWEETS	Yellow cake w/ choc frst,frmix1 cake		3735
SWEETS	Devil's food cake,chocfrst,fmx1 cake		3755
SWEETS	Yellowcake w/ chocfrstng,comml1 cake		3895
SWEETS	Sheetcake,w/ whfrstng,homercip1 cake		4020
SWEETS	White cake w/ wht frstng,comml1 cake		4170
SWEETS	Fruitcake,dark, from homerecip1 cake		5185
SWEETS	Carrot cake,cremchese frst,rec1 cake		6175

CHART BY CARBOHYDRATES

CHART BY CARBOHYDRATES

	Food		Carbohydrate Grams
BEVERAGES	Club soda	12 fl oz	0
BEVERAGES	Coffee, brewed	6 fl oz	0
BEVERAGES	Cola, diet, aspartame only	12 fl oz	0
BEVERAGES	Cola, diet, asprtame + sacchrn	12 fl oz	0
BEVERAGES	Cola, diet, saccharin only	12 fl oz	0
VEGETABLES	Lettuce, butterhead, raw,leave	1 leaf	0
SPICES	Parsley, freeze-dried	1 tbsp	0
SPICES	Salt	1 tsp	0
BEVERAGES	Tea, brewed	8 fl oz	0
SAUCES	Mustard, prepared, yellow	1 tsp	0
DAIRY	Whipped topping, pressurized	1 tbsp	0
DAIRY	Eggs, raw, white	1 white	0
SOUPS	Beef broth, boulln, consm,cnnd	1 cup	0
VEGETABLES	Olives, canned, green	4 medium	0
VEGETABLES	Olives, canned, ripe, mission	3 small	0
MISCELLANEOUS	Gelatin, dry	1 envelp	0
DAIRY	Parmesan cheese, grated	1 tbsp	0
DAIRY	Margarine, spread,hard,60% fat	1 pat	0
POULTRY	Chicken liver, cooked	1 liver	0
DAIRY	Butter, salted	1 pat	0
DAIRY	Butter, unsalted	1 pat	0
DAIRY	Margarine, regulr,hard,80% fat	1 pat	0
POULTRY	Turkey loaf, breast meat w/o c	2 slices	0
POULTRY	Turkey loaf, breast meat, w/ c	2 slices	0
MEATS	Vienna sausage	1 sausag	0
DAIRY	Whipping cream, unwhiped,light	1 tbsp	0
MEATS	Pork, link, cooked	1 link	0
MEATS	Brown and serve sausage,brwnd	1 link	0
DAIRY	Margarine, imitation 40% fat	1 tbsp	0
DAIRY	Whipping cream, unwhiped,heavy	1 tbsp	0
DAIRY	Eggs, raw, yolk	1 yolk	0
DAIRY	Cheddar cheese	1 cu in	0
SAUCES	Vinegar and oil salad dressing	1 tbsp	0
POULTRY	Chicken, roasted, drumstick	1.6 oz	0
POULTRY	Turkey ham, cured turkey thigh	2 slices	0
DAIRY	Margarine, spread,hard,60% fat	1 tbsp	0
DAIRY	Margarine, spread,soft,60% fat	1 tbsp	0

CHART BY CARBOHYDRATES

	Food	Carbohydrate Grams
FISH	Flounder or sole, baked,w/ofat3 oz	0
BEVERAGES	Gin,rum,vodka,whisky 80-proof 1.5 f oz	0
MEATS	Pork, luncheon meat,choppd ham2 slices	0
DAIRY	Butter, salted 1 tbsp	0
DAIRY	Butter, unsalted 1 tbsp	0
DAIRY	Margarine, regulr,hard,80% fat1 tbsp	0
DAIRY	Margarine, regulr,soft,80% fat1 tbsp	0
SAUCES	Mayonnaise, regular 1 tbsp	0
BEVERAGES	Gin,rum,vodka,whisky 86-proof 1.5 f oz	0
MEATS	Pork, cured, ham, rosted,lean 2.4 oz	0
DAIRY	Muenster cheese 1 oz	0
DAIRY	Pasterzd proces cheese,americn1 oz	0
BEVERAGES	Gin,rum,vodka,whisky 90-proof 1.5 f oz	0
MEATS	Pork, cured, bacon, regul,cked3 slice	0
DAIRY	Camembert cheese 1 wedge	0
DAIRY	Cheddar cheese 1 oz	0
SAUCES	Fats, cooking/vegetbl shorteng1 tbsp	0
DAIRY	Lard 1 tbsp	0
FISH	Salmon, canned, pink, w/ bones3 oz	0
FISH	Flounder or sole, baked, buttr3 oz	0
FISH	Flounder or sole, baked,margrn3 oz	0
SAUCES	Corn oil 1 tbsp	0
SAUCES	Olive oil 1 tbsp	0
SAUCES	Peanut oil 1 tbsp	0
OILS	Safflower oil 1 tbsp	0
SAUCES	Soybean oil, hydrogenated 1 tbsp	0
SAUCES	Soybean-cottonseed oil, hydrgn1 tbsp	0
OILS	Sunflower oil 1 tbsp	0
MEATS	Lamb, rib, roasted, lean only 2 oz	0
FISH	Tuna, cannd, drnd,watr, white 3 oz	0
POULTRY	Turkey, roasted, light meat 2 pieces	0
MEATS	Beef roast, eye o rnd, lean 2.6 oz	0
MEATS	Lamb,chops,arm,braised,lean 1.7 oz	0
POULTRY	Chicken, roasted, breast 3.0 oz	0
FISH	Salmon, baked, red 3 oz	0
FISH	Halibut, broiled, butter,lemju3 oz	0
MEATS	Lamb,chops,loin,broil,lean 2.3 oz	0
MEATS	Lamb,leg,roasted, lean only 2.6 oz	0
MEATS	Pork, cured, ham, canned,roast3 oz	0
MEATS	Beef, dried, chipped 2.5 oz	0
POULTRY	Turkey, roasted, light + dark 3 pieces	0

CHART BY CARBOHYDRATES

	Food		Carbohydrate Grams
FISH	Salmon, smoked	3 oz	0
MEATS	Beef roast, rib, lean only	2.2 oz	0
POULTRY	Turkey, roasted, dark meat	4 pieces	0
MEATS	Pork fresh ham, roastd, lean	2.5 oz	0
FISH	Tuna, cannd, drnd,oil,chk,lght3 oz		0
MEATS	Pork chop, loin, broil, lean	2.5 oz	0
MEATS	Pork shoulder, braisd, lean	2.4 oz	0
MEATS	Beef, ckd,chuck blade,leanonly2.2 oz		0
MEATS	Beef, ckd,bttm round,lean only2.8 oz		0
FISH	Sardines, atlntc,cnned,oil,drn3 oz		0
FISH	Trout, broiled, w/ buttr,lemju3 oz		0
MEATS	Pork fresh rib, roastd, lean	2.5 oz	0
MEATS	Pork chop, loin,panfry, lean	2.4 oz	0
MEATS	Veal cutlet, med fat,brsd,brld3 oz		0
MEATS	Beef, canned, corned	3 oz	0
FISH	Herring, pickled	3 oz	0
MEATS	Beef roast, eye o rnd,lean+fat3 oz		0
MEATS	Lamb,leg,roasted, lean+ fat	3 oz	0
MEATS	Pork, cured, ham, rosted,ln+ft3 oz		0
MEATS	Beef, ckd,bttm round,lean+ fat3 oz		0
MEATS	Lamb,chops,arm,braised,lean+ft2.2 oz		0
MEATS	Veal rib, med fat, roasted	3 oz	0
MEATS	Ground beef, broiled, lean	3 oz	0
POULTRY	Chicken, canned, boneless	5 oz	0
MEATS	Lamb,chops,loin,broil,lean+fat2.8 oz		0
POULTRY	Turkey, roasted, light + dark 1 cup		0
MEATS	Beef steak,sirloin,broil,ln+ft3 oz		0
MEATS	Ground beef, broiled, regular 3 oz		0
POULTRY	Chicken, stewed, light + dark 1 cup		0
MEATS	Pork fresh ham, roastd,lean+ft3 oz		0
MEATS	Pork fresh rib, roastd,lean+ft3 oz		0
MEATS	Pork chop, loin, broil, len+ft3.1 oz		0
MEATS	Pork shoulder, braisd,lean+fat3 oz		0
MEATS	Beef roast, rib, lean + fat	3 oz	0
MEATS	Lamb, rib, roasted, lean + fat3 oz		0
MEATS	Beef, ckd,chuck blade,lean+fat3 oz		0
MEATS	Pork chop, loin,panfry,lean+ft3.1 oz		0
POULTRY	Duck, roasted, flesh only	1/2 duck	0
DAIRY	Margarine, spread,hard,60% fat1/2 cup		0
DAIRY	Butter, salted	1/2 cup	0
DAIRY	Butter, unsalted	1/2 cup	0
DAIRY	Margarine, spread,soft,60% fat8 oz		0

CHART BY CARBOHYDRATES

	Food		Carbohydrate Grams
SAUCES	Olive oil	1 cup	0
SAUCES	Peanut oil	1 cup	0
SAUCES	Corn oil	1 cup	0
OILS	Safflower oil	1 cup	0
SAUCES	Soybean oil, hydrogenated	1 cup	0
SAUCES	Soybean-cottonseed oil, hydrgn	1 cup	0
OILS	Sunflower oil	1 cup	0
BEVERAGES	Coffee, instant, prepared	6 fl oz	1
BEVERAGES	Tea, instant,preprd,unsweetend	8 fl oz	1
SAUCES	Vinegar, cider	1 tbsp	1
MISCELLANEOUS	Baking powder, low sodium	1 tsp	1
MISCELLANEOUS	Baking powder, strght phosphat	1 tsp	1
MISCELLANEOUS	Baking powder,sas, ca po4	1 tsp	1
BREADS	Baking powder,sas,capo4+caso4	1 tsp	1
VEGETABLES	Celery, pascal type, raw,stalk	1 stalk	1
VEGETABLES	Cucumber, w/ peel	6 slices	1
SPICES	Curry powder	1 tsp	1
FRUITS	Lemon juice, canned	1 tbsp	1
VEGETABLES	Lettuce, crisphead, raw,pieces	1 cup	1
SPICES	Oregano	1 tsp	1
SPICES	Paprika	1 tsp	1
VEGETABLES	Parsley, raw	10 sprig	1
SPICES	Pepper, black	1 tsp	1
VEGETABLES	Pickles, cucumber, dill	1 pickle	1
VEGETABLES	Radishes, raw	4 radish	1
VEGETABLES	Alfalfa seeds, sprouted, raw	1 cup	1
SPICES	Chili powder	1 tsp	1
DAIRY	Imitatn whipd toping,pwdrd,prp	1 tbsp	1
SPICES	Celery seed	1 tsp	1
DAIRY	Imitation creamers, powdered	1 tsp	1
DAIRY	Imitatn whipd toping,pressrzd	1 tbsp	1
SOUPS	Bouillon, dehydrtd, unprepared	1 pkt	1
DAIRY	Imitation whipped topping,frzn	1 tbsp	1
BEVERAGES	Half and half, cream	1 tbsp	1
DAIRY	Imitatn sour dressing	1 tbsp	1
DAIRY	Sour cream	1 tbsp	1
DAIRY	Light, coffee or table cream	1 tbsp	1
SPICES	Sesame seeds	1 tbsp	1
MEATS	Pork, luncheon meat,ckd ham,ln	2 slices	1
DAIRY	Eggs, cooked, hard-cooked	1 egg	1
DAIRY	Eggs, cooked, poached	1 egg	1
DAIRY	Eggs, raw, whole	1 egg	1

CHART BY CARBOHYDRATES

	Food		Carbohydrate Grams
SAUCES	Tartar sauce	1 tbsp	1
DAIRY	Mozzarella chese,skim, lomoist	1 oz	1
DAIRY	Mozzarella cheese, whole milk	1 oz	1
SAUCES	Italian salad dressing,regular	1 tbsp	1
MEATS	Pork, cured, bacon,canadn,cked	2 slice	1
MEATS	Salami, dry type	2 slices	1
SAUCES	French salad dressing, regular	1 tbsp	1
POULTRY	Chicken roll, light	2 slices	1
DAIRY	Eggs, cooked, fried	1 egg	1
DAIRY	Pasterzd proces cheese, swiss	1 oz	1
FISH	Shrimp, canned, drained	3 oz	1
DAIRY	Eggs, cooked, scrambled/omelet	1 egg	1
DAIRY	Blue cheese	1 oz	1
DAIRY	Provolone cheese	1 oz	1
DAIRY	Cream cheese	1 oz	1
DAIRY	Swiss cheese	1 oz	1
POULTRY	Chicken, fried, flour, drmstck	1.7 oz	1
DAIRY	Parmesan cheese, grated	1 oz	1
FISH	Crabmeat, canned	1 cup	1
MEATS	Pork, luncheon meat,canned	2 slices	1
MEATS	Salami, cooked type	2 slices	1
MEATS	Frankfurter, cooked	1 frank	1
DAIRY	Chedddar cheese, shredded	1 cup	1
DAIRY	Margarine, imitation 40% fat	8 oz	1
DAIRY	Margarine, regulr,hard,80% fat	1/2 cup	1
DAIRY	Margarine, regulr,soft,80% fat	8 oz	1
SPICES	Cinnamon	1 tsp	2
SAUCES	Italian salad dressing,localor	1 tbsp	2
SPICES	Onion powder	1 tsp	2
VEGETABLES	Asparagus,canned,spears,nosalt	4 spears	2
VEGETABLES	Asparagus,canned,spears,w/salt	4 spears	2
SAUCES	Barbecue sauce	1 tbsp	2
VEGETABLES	Broccoli, frzn, cooked, draned	1 piece	2
VEGETABLES	Cabbage, chinese,pe-tsai, raw	1 cup	2
VEGETABLES	Endive, curly, raw	1 cup	2
SPICES	Garlic powder	1 tsp	2
VEGETABLES	Lettuce, looseleaf	1 cup	2
VEGETABLES	Onions, spring, raw	6 onion	2
BREADS	Pretzels, stick	10 pretz	2
SAUCES	Soy sauce	1 tbsp	2
VEGETABLES	Spinach, raw	1 cup	2
BREADS	Snack type crackers	1 crackr	2

CHART BY CARBOHYDRATES

	Food	Carbohydrate Grams
SAUCES	Cooked salad drssing, home rcp1 tbsp	2
SAUCES	French salad dressing, localor1 tbsp	2
SAUCES	Mayonnaise, imitation 1 tbsp	2
BREADS	Sandwich spread, pork, beef 1 tbsp	2
SAUCES	1000 island, salad drsng,reglr1 tbsp	2
FISH	Clams, raw 3 oz	2
DAIRY	Pasterzd proces chese spred,am1 oz	2
FISH	Clams, canned, drained 3 oz	2
DAIRY	Pasterzd proces chese food,amr1 oz	2
MEATS	Pork, luncheon meat,ckd ham,rg2 slices	2
MEATS	Bologna 2 slices	2
MEATS	Braunschweiger 2 slices	2
POULTRY	Chicken, fried, flour, breast 3.5 oz	2
VEGETABLES	Pickles, cucumber, fresh pack 2 slices	3
VEGETABLES	Seaweed, kelp, raw 1 oz	3
VEGETABLES	Asparagus, ckd frm frz,dr,sper4 spears	3
VEGETABLES	Asparagus, ckd frm raw,dr,sper4 spears	3
VEGETABLES	Peppers, sweet, cooked, green 1 pepper	3
VEGETABLES	Peppers, sweet, cooked, red 1 pepper	3
VEGETABLES	Cabbage, chinese, pak-choi,ckd1 cup	3
VEGETABLES	Lettuce, crisphead, raw,wedge 1 wedge	3
VEGETABLES	Mushrooms, raw 1 cup	3
VEGETABLES	Mustard greens, cooked, draned1 cup	3
MISCELLANEOUS	Yeast, bakers, dry, active 1 pkg	3
MISCELLANEOUS	Yeast, brewers, dry 1 tbsp	3
BEVERAGES	Wine, table, red 3.5 f oz	3
BEVERAGES	Wine, table, white 3.5 f oz	3
DAIRY	Tofu 1 piece	3
NUTS	Peanut butter 1 tbsp	3
POULTRY	Chicken frankfurter 1 frank	3
DAIRY	Cottage cheese,uncreamed 1 cup	3
POULTRY	Turkey roast, frzn,lght+drk,ck3 oz	3
NUTS	Walnuts, black, chopped 1 oz	3
VEGETABLES	Spinach souffle 1 cup	3
VEGETABLES	Cabbage, common, raw 1 cup	4
SAUCES	Catsup 1 tbsp	4
FRUITS	Plums, raw, 1-1/2-in diam 1 plum	4
VEGETABLES	Cabbage, red, raw 1 cup	4
VEGETABLES	Cabbage, savoy, raw 1 cup	4
VEGETABLES	Celery, pascal type, raw,piece1 cup	4
VEGETABLES	Lettuce, butterhead, raw,head 1 head	4
BREADS	Melba toast, plain 1 piece	4

CHART BY CARBOHYDRATES

	Food	Carbohydrate Grams
VEGETABLES	Peppers, hot chili, raw, green 1 pepper	4
VEGETABLES	Peppers, hot chili, raw, red 1 pepper	4
VEGETABLES	Peppers, sweet, raw, green 1 pepper	4
VEGETABLES	Peppers, sweet, raw, red 1 pepper	4
VEGETABLES	Bamboo shoots, canned, drained 1 cup	4
SAUCES	Mayonnaise type salad dressing 1 tbsp	4
FISH	Fish sticks, frozen, reheated 1 stick	4
NUTS	Filberts, (hazelnuts) chopped 1 oz	4
NUTS	Brazil nuts 1 oz	4
NUTS	Macadamia nuts, oilrstd,salted 1 oz	4
NUTS	Macadamia nuts, oilrstd,unsalt 1 oz	4
DAIRY	Parmesan cheese, grated 1 cup	4
FRUITS	Lemons, raw 1 lemon	5
VEGETABLES	Pickles, cucumber, swt gherkin 1 pickle	5
SAUCES	Relish, sweet 1 tbsp	5
VEGETABLES	Bean sprouts, mung, cookd,dran 1 cup	5
VEGETABLES	Cauliflower, raw 1 cup	5
VEGETABLES	Collards, cooked from raw 1 cup	5
VEGETABLES	Tomatoes, raw 1 tomato	5
BREADS	Wheat, thin crackers 4 crackr	5
SWEETS	Whole-wheat wafers, crackers 2 crackr	5
BREADS	Cheese crackers, sandwch,peant 1 sandwh	5
FISH	Oysters, breaded, fried 1 oyster	5
BEVERAGES	Beer, light 12 fl oz	5
VEGETABLES	Pumpkin and squash kernels 1 oz	5
NUTS	Sunflower seeds 1 oz	5
NUTS	Pine nuts 1 oz	5
NUTS	Peanuts, oil roasted, salted 1 oz	5
NUTS	Peanuts, oil roasted, unsalted 1 oz	5
NUTS	Walnuts, english, pieces 1 oz	5
NUTS	Pecans, halves 1 oz	5
VEGETABLES	Eggplant, cooked, steamed 1 cup	6
VEGETABLES	Okra pods, cooked 8 pods	6
VEGETABLES	Snap bean,cnnd,drnd,green,salt 1 cup	6
VEGETABLES	Snap bean,cnnd,drnd,grn,nosalt 1 cup	6
VEGETABLES	Snap bean,cnnd,drnd,yllw, salt 1 cup	6
VEGETABLES	Snap bean,cnnd,drnd,yllw,nosal 1 cup	6
SWEETS	Sugar, white, granulated 1 pkt	6
VEGETABLES	Bean sprouts, mung, raw 1 cup	6
VEGETABLES	Cauliflower, cooked from raw 1 cup	6
NUTS	Popcorn, air-popped, unsalted 1 cup	6
VEGETABLES	Turnip greens, cooked from raw 1 cup	6

CHART BY CARBOHYDRATES

	Food	Carbohydrate Grams
BREADS	Pancakes, buckwheat, from mix 1 pancak	6
NUTS	Popcorn, popped, veg oil,saltd1 cup	6
NUTS	Almonds, whole 1 oz	6
NUTS	Mixed nuts w/ peants,oil,saltd1 oz	6
NUTS	Mixed nuts w/ peants,oil,unslt1 oz	6
POULTRY	Chicken, fried, batter,drmstck2.5 oz	6
DAIRY	Cottage cheese,cremd,smll curd1 cup	6
DAIRY	Cottage cheese,cremd,lrge curd1 cup	6
VEGETABLES	Beets, cooked, drained, whole 2 beets	7
VEGETABLES	Cabbage, common, cooked, drned1 cup	7
VEGETABLES	Carrots, raw, whole 1 carrot	7
VEGETABLES	Cauliflower, cooked from frozn1 cup	7
VEGETABLES	Dandelion greens, cooked, drnd1 cup	7
VEGETABLES	Spinach, cooked from raw, drnd1 cup	7
VEGETABLES	Kale, cooked from frozen 1 cup	7
VEGETABLES	Kale, cooked from raw 1 cup	7
VEGETABLES	Spinach, canned, drnd,w/ salt 1 cup	7
VEGETABLES	Spinach, canned, drnd,w/o salt1 cup	7
SOUPS	Chicken rice soup, canned 1 cup	7
VEGETABLES	Seaweed, spirulina, dried 1 oz	7
SAUCES	Gravy and turkey, frozen 5 oz	7
DAIRY	Whipped topping, pressurized 1 cup	7
SWEETS	Coconut, raw, piece 1 piece	7
NUTS	Pistachio nuts 1 oz	7
NUTS	Mixed nuts w/ peants,dry,saltd1 oz	7
NUTS	Mixed nuts w/ peants,dry,unslt1 oz	7
FISH	Haddock, breaded, fried 3 oz	7
MEATS	Beef liver, fried 3 oz	7
FISH	Ocean perch, breaded, fried 1 fillet	7
DAIRY	Ricotta cheese, whole milk 1 cup	7
DAIRY	Whipping cream, unwhiped,light1 cup	7
DAIRY	Whipping cream, unwhiped,heavy1 cup	7
VEGETABLES	Turnips, cooked, diced 1 cup	8
VEGETABLES	Carrots, canned, drn, w/ salt 1 cup	8
VEGETABLES	Carrots, canned,drnd, w/o salt1 cup	8
VEGETABLES	Mushrooms, canned, drnd,w/salt1 cup	8
VEGETABLES	Snap bean,frz,ckd,drnd,green 1 cup	8
VEGETABLES	Snap bean,frz,ckd,drnd,yellow 1 cup	8
VEGETABLES	Sweetpotatoes, cnned, vac pack1 piece	8
VEGETABLES	Squash, summer, cooked, draind1 cup	8
VEGETABLES	Beet greens, cooked, drained 1 cup	8
VEGETABLES	Onions, raw, sliced 1 cup	8

CHART BY CARBOHYDRATES

	Food	Carbohydrate Grams
SOUPS	Tomato veg soup, dehyd,prepred1 pkt	8
VEGETABLES	Asparagus, ckd frm raw, dr,cut1 cup	8
VEGETABLES	Turnip greens, cked frm frozen1 cup	8
BREADS	Pancakes, plain, from mix 1 pancak	8
VEGETABLES	Onion rings, breaded,frzn,prpd2 rings	8
BEVERAGES	Wine, dessert 3.5 f oz	8
SWEETS	Chocolate, bitter ot baking 1 oz	8
FISH	Oysters, raw 1 cup	8
NUTS	Cashew nuts, oil roastd,salted1 oz	8
NUTS	Cashew nuts, oil roastd,unsalt1 oz	8
DAIRY	Cottage cheese,lowfat 2% 1 cup	8
FRUITS	Grapes, european, raw, thompsn10 grape	9
FRUITS	Peaches, canned, juice pack 1 half	9
FRUITS	Pineapple, canned, juice pack 1 slice	9
FRUITS	Plums, raw, 2-1/8-in diam 1 plum	9
FRUITS	Tangerines, raw 1 tangrn	9
VEGETABLES	Broccoli, raw, cooked, drained1 cup	9
VEGETABLES	Asparagus, ckd frm frz,drn,cut1 cup	9
BREADS	Saltines 4 crackr	9
BREADS	Pancakes, plain, home recipe 1 pancak	9
SOUPS	Chicken noodle soup, canned 1 cup	9
SOUPS	Beef noodle soup, canned 1 cup	9
SOUPS	Cr of chicken soup w/ h20,cnnd1 cup	9
SOUPS	Cr of mushrom soup w/ h2o,cnnd1 cup	9
NUTS	Cashew nuts, dry roastd,salted1 oz	9
NUTS	Cashew nuts, dry roastd,unsalt1 oz	9
DAIRY	Light, coffee or table cream 1 cup	9
FRUITS	Peaches, raw 1 peach	10
FRUITS	Apricots, canned, juice pack 3 halves	10
BEVERAGES	Grapefruit, raw, pink 1/2 frut	10
BEVERAGES	Grapefruit, raw, white 1/2 frut	10
FRUITS	Grapes, european, raw, tokay 10 grape	10
FRUITS	Jams and preserves 1 pkt	10
FRUITS	Jellies 1 pkt	10
FRUITS	Pears, canned, juice pack 1 half	10
BEVERAGES	Tomato juice, canned w/o salt 1 cup	10
BEVERAGES	Tomato juice, canned with salt1 cup	10
VEGETABLES	Sauerkraut, canned 1 cup	10
VEGETABLES	Snap bean,raw,ckd,drnd,green 1 cup	10
VEGETABLES	Snap bean,raw,ckd,drnd,yellow 1 cup	10
FRUITS	Strawberries, raw 1 cup	10
VEGETABLES	Broccoli, frzn, cooked, draned1 cup	10

CHART BY CARBOHYDRATES

	Food	Carbohydrate Grams
VEGETABLES	Tomatoes, canned, s+l,w/o salt1 cup	10
VEGETABLES	Spinach, cooked fr frzen, drnd1 cup	10
BREADS	Rye wafers, whole-grain 2 wafers	10
BREADS	White bread, slice 22 per loaf1 slice	10
BREADS	White bread, toasted 22 per 1 slice	10
BREADS	Baking pwdr biscuits,refrgdogh1 biscut	10
SOUPS	Vegetable beef soup, canned 1 cup	10
BREADS	Potato chips 10 chips	10
POULTRY	Turkey patties, brd,battd,frid1 patty	10
FISH	Scallops, breaded, frzn,reheat6 scalop	10
POULTRY	Chicken chow mein, home recipe1 cup	10
BEVERAGES	Half and half, cream 1 cup	10
DAIRY	Sour cream 1 cup	10
FRUITS	Raisins 1 packet	11
VEGETABLES	Carrots, raw, grated 1 cup	11
FRUITS	Kiwifruit, raw 1 kiwi	11
BEVERAGES	Vegetable juice cocktail, cnnd1 cup	11
FRUITS	Cherries, sweet, raw 10 chery	11
FRUITS	Watermelon, raw, diced 1 cup	11
VEGETABLES	Beets, cooked, drained, diced 1 cup	11
SWEETS	Graham cracker, plain 2 crackr	11
VEGETABLES	Peas, edible pod, cooked,drned1 cup	11
VEGETABLES	Lettuce, crisphead, raw, head 1 head	11
SOUPS	Minestrone soup, canned 1 cup	11
SWEETS	Brownies w/ nuts,frm home recp1 browne	11
SAUCES	Beef gravy, canned 1 cup	11
DAIRY	Yogurt, w/ whole milk 8 oz	11
DAIRY	Milk, whole, 3.3% fat 1 cup	11
DAIRY	Imitatn whipd toping,pressrzd 1 cup	11
FISH	Shrimp, french fried 3 oz	11
DAIRY	Imitatn sour dressing 1 cup	11
FRUITS	Honeydew melon, raw 1/10 mel	12
FRUITS	Pineapple, canned, heavy syrup1 slice	12
SWEETS	Sugar, white, granulated 1 tbsp	12
FRUITS	Apricots, raw 3 aprcot	12
VEGETABLES	Pumpkin, cooked from raw 1 cup	12
VEGETABLES	Artichokes, globe, cooked, drn1 artchk	12
VEGETABLES	Beets, canned, drained,no salt1 cup	12
VEGETABLES	Beets, canned, drained,w/ salt1 cup	12
VEGETABLES	Carrots, cooked from frozen 1 cup	12
VEGETABLES	Onions, raw, chopped 1 cup	12
VEGETABLES	Collards, cooked from frozen 1 cup	12

CHART BY CARBOHYDRATES

	Food	Carbohydrate Grams
BREADS	Mixed grain bread 1 slice	12
BREADS	Mixed grain bread, toasted 1 slice	12
BREADS	Oatmeal bread 1 slice	12
BREADS	Oatmeal bread, toasted 1 slice	12
BREADS	Rye bread, light 1 slice	12
BREADS	Rye bread, light, toasted 1 slice	12
BREADS	Wheat bread 1 slice	12
BREADS	Wheat bread, toasted 1 slice	12
BREADS	White bread, slice 18 per loaf1 slice	12
BREADS	White bread, toasted 18 per 1 slice	12
SOUPS	Vegetarian soup, canned 1 cup	12
SOUPS	Clam chowder, manhattan, cannd1 cup	12
DAIRY	Milk, skim, no added milksolid1 cup	12
DAIRY	Milk, skim, added milk solids 1 cup	12
DAIRY	Buttermilk, fluid 1 cup	12
DAIRY	Milk, lofat, 1%, no addedsolid1 cup	12
DAIRY	Ice cream, vanlla, regulr 11% 3 fl oz	12
DAIRY	Milk, lofat, 1%, added solids 1 cup	12
DAIRY	Milk, lofat, 2%, no addedsolid1 cup	12
DAIRY	Milk, lofat, 2%, added solids 1 cup	12
SWEETS	Coconut, raw, shredded 1 cup	12
VEGETABLES	Avocados, california 1 avocdo	12
POULTRY	Chicken a la king, home recipe1 cup	12
FRUITS	Jellies 1 tbsp	13
VEGETABLES	Onions, raw, cooked, drained 1 cup	13
VEGETABLES	Brussels sprouts, raw, cooked 1 cup	13
VEGETABLES	Brussels sprouts, frzn, cooked1 cup	13
BREADS	Pretzels, twisted, dutch 1 pretz	13
BREADS	Raisin bread 1 slice	13
BREADS	Raisin bread, toasted 1 slice	13
BREADS	Tortillas, corn 1 tortla	13
BREADS	Vienna bread 1 slice	13
SWEETS	Whole-wheat bread 1 slice	13
SWEETS	Whole-wheat bread, toasted 1 slice	13
BREADS	Baking pwdr biscuits,homerecpe1 biscut	13
BREADS	Danish pastry, plain, no nuts 1 oz	13
SAUCES	Mushroom gravy, canned 1 cup	13
BEVERAGES	Beer, regular 12 fl oz	13
DAIRY	Imitatn whipd toping,pwdrd,prp1 cup	13
SWEETS	Milk chocolate candy,w/ penuts1 oz	13
SAUCES	Chicken gravy, canned 1 cup	13
MEATS	Chop suey w/ beef + pork,hmrcp1 cup	13

CHART BY CARBOHYDRATES

	Food	Carbohydrate Grams
FRUITS	Jams and preserves 1 tbsp	14
FRUITS	Plums, canned, juice pack 3 plums	14
VEGETABLES	Corn, cooked frm frozn, white 1 ear	14
VEGETABLES	Corn, cooked frm frozn, yellow1 ear	14
FRUITS	Raspberries, raw 1 cup	14
SAUCES	Brown gravy from dry mix 1 cup	14
SAUCES	Chicken gravy from dry mix 1 cup	14
BREADS	Rolls, dinner, commercial 1 roll	14
BREADS	Baking pwdr biscuits,from mix 1 biscut	14
SAUCES	Hollandaise sce, w/ h2o,frm mx1 cup	14
FRUITS	Oranges, raw 1 orange	15
FRUITS	Pears, canned, heavy syrup 1 half	15
VEGETABLES	Vegetables, mixed, canned 1 cup	15
BREADS	White bread cubes 1 cup	15
DAIRY	Malted milk,natural, powder 3/4 oz	15
SWEETS	Pound cake, commercial 1 slice	15
SWEETS	Pound cake, from home recipe 1 slice	15
SWEETS	Milk chocolate candy,w/ almond1 oz	15
SOUPS	Cr of chicken soup w/ mlk,cnnd1 cup	15
BREADS	Taco 1 taco	15
SOUPS	Cr of mushrom soup w/ mlk,cnnd1 cup	15
MEATS	Beef and vegetable stew,hm rcp1 cup	15
NUTS	Walnuts, black, chopped 1 cup	15
FRUITS	Lemon juice, canned 1 cup	16
FRUITS	Lime juice,canned 1 cup	16
BEVERAGES	Lemon juice,frzn,single-strngh6 fl oz	16
FRUITS	Peaches, canned, heavy syrup 1 half	16
FRUITS	Apples, raw, peeled, sliced 1 cup	16
FRUITS	Nectarines, raw 1 nectrn	16
VEGETABLES	Carrots, cooked from raw 1 cup	16
BREADS	Pumpernickel bread 1 slice	16
BREADS	Pumpernickel bread, toasted 1 slice	16
SWEETS	Brownies w/ nuts,frstng,cmmrcl1 browne	16
DAIRY	Yogurt, w/ lofat milk, plain 8 oz	16
SWEETS	Milk chocolate candy, plain 1 oz	16
SWEETS	Sweet (dark) chocolate 1 oz	16
BREADS	Corn chips 1 oz	16
SWEETS	Honey 1 tbsp	17
FRUITS	Papayas, raw 1 cup	17
MISCELLANEOUS	Gelatin dessert, prepared 1/2 cup	17
NUTS	Water chestnuts, canned 1 cup	17
BREADS	Italian bread 1 slice	17

CHART BY CARBOHYDRATES

	Food	Carbohydrate Grams
VEGETABLES	Potatoes,french-frd,frzn,oven 10 strip	17
DAIRY	Yogurt, w/ nonfat milk 8 oz	17
SWEETS	Shortbread cookie, home recipe2 cookie	17
BREADS	French toast, home recipe 1 slice	17
SOUPS	Clam chowder, new eng, w/ milk1 cup	17
DAIRY	Imitation whipped topping,frzn1 cup	17
NUTS	Macadamia nuts, oilrstd,salted1 cup	17
NUTS	Macadamia nuts, oilrstd,unsalt1 cup	17
FRUITS	Apricot, canned, heavy syrup 3 halves	18
SAUCES	Tomato sauce, canned with salt1 cup	18
FRUITS	Blackberries, raw 1 cup	18
BREADS	Corn grits, cooked, instant 1 pkt	18
VEGETABLES	Squash, winter, baked 1 cup	18
DAIRY	Malted milk, chocolate, powder3/4 oz	18
POULTRY	Chicken chow mein, canned 1 cup	18
BREADS	French bread 1 slice	18
BREADS	Oatmeal,ckd,instnt,plain,fortf1 pkt	18
CEREAL	100% natural cereal 1 oz	18
SWEETS	Milk chocolate candy,w/ rice c1 oz	18
SWEETS	Popsicle 1 popcle	18
NUTS	Filberts, (hazelnuts) chopped 1 cup	18
FRUITS	Peaches, raw, sliced 1 cup	19
SWEETS	Coca pwdr w/o nonfat dry milk 3/4 oz	19
FRUITS	Pineapple, raw, diced 1 cup	19
VEGETABLES	Corn, cooked from raw, white 1 ear	19
VEGETABLES	Corn, cooked from raw, yellow 1 ear	19
CEREAL	Nature valley granola cereal 1 oz	19
BREADS	Bran muffins, home recipe 1 muffin	19
SAUCES	Soybeans, dry, cooked, drained1 cup	19
FISH	Tuna salad 1 cup	19
BEVERAGES	Limeade,concen,frozen,diluted 6 fl oz	20
FRUITS	Blueberries, raw 1 cup	20
VEGETABLES	Pumpkin, canned 1 cup	20
CEREAL	Cheerios cereal 1 oz	20
BREADS	Rolls, frankfurter + hamburger1 roll	20
BREADS	Rolls, dinner, home recipe 1 roll	20
SWEETS	Devil's food cake,chocfrst,fmx1 cupcak	20
SWEETS	Blueberry muffins, home recipe1 muffin	20
VEGETABLES	Potatoes,french-frd,frzn,fried10 strip	20
NUTS	Pecans, halves 1 cup	20
SWEETS	Shortbread cookie, commercial 4 cookie	20
FRUITS	Lemon juice, raw 1 cup	21

CHART BY CARBOHYDRATES

	Food	Carbohydrate Grams
BEVERAGES	Lemonade,concen,frzen,diluted 6 fl oz	21
FRUITS	Oranges, raw, sections 1 cup	21
FRUITS	Pears, raw, bosc 1 pear	21
CEREAL	Raisin bran, post 1 oz	21
CEREAL	Raisin bran, kellogg's 1 oz	21
BREADS	Boston brown bread,w/whtecrnm 1 slice	21
BREADS	Boston brown bread,w/yllwcrnml1 slice	21
DAIRY	Cream of wheat,ckd,mix n eat 1 pkt	21
CEREAL	Special K cereal 1 oz	21
VEGETABLES	Peas, green,cnnd,drnd, w/ salt1 cup	21
VEGETABLES	Peas, green,cnnd,drnd,w/o salt1 cup	21
SWEETS	Fudge, chocolate, plain 1 oz	21
SWEETS	Syrup, chocolate flvred, fudge2 tbsp	21
SWEETS	White sauce w/ milk from mix 1 cup	21
FRUITS	Lime juice, raw 1 cup	22
BEVERAGES	Fruit punch drink, canned 6 fl oz	22
SWEETS	Molasses, cane, blackstrap 2 tbsp	22
SWEETS	Syrup, chocolate flavored thin2 tbsp	22
BEVERAGES	Tea,instant,prepard,sweetened 8 fl oz	22
CEREAL	Bran flakes, post 1 oz	22
FRUITS	Cherries, sour,red,cannd,water1 cup	22
CEREAL	Bran flakes, kellogg's 1 oz	22
BEVERAGES	Grapefruit juice, canned,unswt1 cup	22
FRUITS	Cantaloup, raw 1/2 meln	22
SWEETS	Cocoa pwdr w/ nofat drmlk,prpd1 servng	22
SWEETS	Cocoa pwdr with nonfat drymilk1 oz	22
CEREAL	Total cereal 1 oz	22
SWEETS	Caramels, plain or chocolate 1 oz	22
BREADS	White bread crumbs, soft 1 cup	22
SWEETS	Blueberry muffins,from com mix1 muffin	22
BREADS	Corn muffins, from commerl mix1 muffin	22
SOUPS	Tomato soup with milk, canned 1 cup	22
NUTS	Walnuts, english, pieces 1 cup	22
SWEETS	Marshmallows 1 oz	23
BEVERAGES	Pineapple-grapefruit juicedrnk6 fl oz	23
BEVERAGES	Grapefruit juice, raw 1 cup	23
CEREAL	Grape-nuts cereal 1 oz	23
CEREAL	Wheaties cereal 1 oz	23
CEREAL	Shredded wheat cereal 1 oz	23
CEREAL	Honey nut cheerios cereal 1 oz	23
BREADS	Lucky charms cereal 1 oz	23
CEREAL	Cap'n crunch cereal 1 oz	23

CHART BY CARBOHYDRATES

	Food	Carbohydrate Grams
DAIRY	Cheese sauce w/ milk, frm mix 1 cup	23
BEVERAGES	Grapefrt jce,frzn,dltd,unswten1 cup	24
VEGETABLES	Vegetables, mixed, cked fr frz1 cup	24
CEREAL	Corn flakes, kellogg's 1 oz	24
CEREAL	Corn flakes, toasties 1 oz	24
CEREAL	Product 19 cereal 1 oz	24
CEREAL	Golden grahams cereal 1 oz	24
PASTA	Macaroni, cooked, tender,cold 1 cup	24
BREADS	Bran muffins, from commerl mix1 muffin	24
SWEETS	Doughnuts, cake type, plain 1 donut	24
BREADS	Enchilada 1 enchld	24
SWEETS	White sauce, medium, home recp1 cup	24
SWEETS	Gum drops 1 oz	25
FRUITS	Pears, raw, bartlett 1 pear	25
BEVERAGES	Orange + grapefruit juce,cannd1 cup	25
BEVERAGES	Orange juice, canned 1 cup	25
SAUCES	Tomato puree, canned w/o salt 1 cup	25
SAUCES	Tomato puree, canned with salt1 cup	25
CEREAL	Sugar smacks cereal 1 oz	25
BREADS	Rice krispies cereal 1 oz	25
CEREAL	Trix cereal 1 oz	25
CEREAL	Froot loops cereal 1 oz	25
BEVERAGES	Orange juice, chilled 1 cup	25
BREADS	Oatmeal,ckd,rg,qck,inst,w/osal1 cup	25
BREADS	Oatmeal,ckd,rg,qck,inst,w/salt1 cup	25
DAIRY	Pudding, tapioca, from mix 1/2 cup	25
DAIRY	Pudding, vnlla,cooked from mix1/2 cup	25
DAIRY	Pudding, choc, cooked from mix1/2 cup	25
SWEETS	Fruitcake,dark, from homerecip1 piece	25
BEVERAGES	Evaporated milk, whole, canned1 cup	25
BEVERAGES	Grape drink, canned 6 fl oz	26
SWEETS	Jelly beans 1 oz	26
CEREAL	Super sugar crisp cereal 1 oz	26
BEVERAGES	Orange juice, raw 1 cup	26
CEREAL	Sugar frosted flakes, kellogg 1 oz	26
VEGETABLES	Jerusalem-artichoke, raw 1 cup	26
BREADS	Cornmeal,degermed,enrched,cook1 cup	26
BEVERAGES	Chocolate milk, lowfat 1% 1 cup	26
BEVERAGES	Chocolate milk, lowfat 2% 1 cup	26
SWEETS	Chocolate chip cookies,hme rcp4 cookie	26
BEVERAGES	Chocolate milk, regular 1 cup	26
VEGETABLES	Potatoes, scalloped, home recp1 cup	26

CHART BY CARBOHYDRATES

	Food	Carbohydrate Grams
PASTA	Macaroni and cheese, canned 1 cup	26
SWEETS	Doughnuts, yeast-leavend,glzed1 donut	26
BREADS	Waffles, from home recipe 1 waffle	26
SWEETS	Cheesecake 1 piece	26
POULTRY	Chicken and noodles, home recp1 cup	26
FRUITS	Bananas 1 banana	27
BEVERAGES	Orange juice,frzn,cncn,diluted1 cup	27
VEGETABLES	Potatoes, boiled, peeled befor1 potato	27
VEGETABLES	Potatoes, boiled, peeled after1 potato	27
BREADS	English muffins, plain 1 muffin	27
BREADS	English muffins, plain, toastd1 muffin	27
DAIRY	Pudding, vnlla,instant frm mix1/2 cup	27
DAIRY	Pudding, choc, instant, fr mix1/2 cup	27
DAIRY	Pudding, rice, from mix 1/2 cup	27
SWEETS	Snack cakes,sponge creme fllngsm cake	27
SOUPS	Pea, green, soup, canned 1 cup	27
BREADS	Waffles, from mix 1 waffle	27
DAIRY	Malted milk,natural, pwdr pprd1 servng	27
BREADS	Croissants 1 crosst	27
VEGETABLES	Avocados, florida 1 avocdo	27
NUTS	Peanuts, oil roasted, salted 1 cup	27
NUTS	Peanuts, oil roasted, unsalted1 cup	27
FRUITS	Applesauce, canned,unsweetened1 cup	28
SWEETS	Hard candy 1 oz	28
BEVERAGES	Grapefruit juice, canned,swtnd1 cup	28
VEGETABLES	Sweetpotatoes, baked, peeled 1 potato	28
DAIRY	Pudding, tapioca, canned 5 oz	28
SWEETS	Chocolate chip cookies,commrcl4 cookie	28
BREADS	Danish pastry, fruit 1 pastry	28
MEATS	Hamburger, regular 1 sandwh	28
NUTS	Peanut butter cookie,home recp4 cookie	28
MEATS	Cheeseburger, regular 1 sandwh	28
VEGETABLES	Potatoes, au gratin, home recp1 cup	28
VEGETABLES	Potato salad made w/ mayonnais1 cup	28
NUTS	Almonds, slivered 1 cup	28
FRUITS	Peaches, canned, juice pack 1 cup	29
BEVERAGES	Apple juice, canned 1 cup	29
FRUITS	Fruit cocktail,cnnd,juice pack1 cup	29
SWEETS	Angelfood cake, from mix 1 piece	29
DAIRY	Crm wheat,ckd, quick, no salt 1 cup	29
DAIRY	Crm wheat,ckd,quick, w/ salt 1 cup	29
DAIRY	Crm wheat,ckd,reg,inst,no salt1 cup	29

CHART BY CARBOHYDRATES

	Food	Carbohydrate Grams
DAIRY	Ice milk, vanilla, 4% fat 1 cup	29
SWEETS	Vanilla wafers 10 cooke	29
SWEETS	Sandwich type cookie 4 cookie	29
BEVERAGES	Evaporated milk, skim, canned 1 cup	29
DAIRY	Malted milk,chocolate, pwdrppd1 servng	29
PASTA	Spaghetti,meatballs,tomsac,cnd1 cup	29
SWEETS	Custard, baked 1 cup	29
DAIRY	Quiche lorraine 1 slice	29
FRUITS	Pears, raw, d'anjou 1 pear	30
VEGETABLES	Parsnips, cooked, drained 1 cup	30
FRUITS	Tangerine juice, canned,swtned1 cup	30
NUTS	Popcorn, sugar syrup coated 1 cup	30
BREADS	Rolls, hard 1 roll	30
VEGETABLES	Blackeye peas, immatr,raw,cked1 cup	30
DAIRY	Pudding, chocolate,canned 5 oz	30
SWEETS	Coca pwdr w/o nofat drymlk,prd1 servng	30
DAIRY	Cottage cheese,cremd,w/fruit 1 cup	30
FRUITS	Prunes, dried 5 large	31
FRUITS	Apricots, canned, juice pack 1 cup	31
FRUITS	Plums, canned, heavy syrup 3 plums	31
BREADS	Corn grits,ckd,reg,whte,nosalt1 cup	31
BREADS	Corn grits,ckd,reg,whte,w/salt1 cup	31
BREADS	Corn grits,ckd,reg,yllw,nosalt1 cup	31
BREADS	Corn grits,ckd,reg,yllw,w/salt1 cup	31
BREADS	Oatmeal,ckd,instnt,flvrd,fortf1 pkt	31
VEGETABLES	Potatoes, au gratin, from mix 1 cup	31
VEGETABLES	Potatoes, scalloped, from mix 1 cup	31
SWEETS	Sugar cookie, from refrig dogh4 cookie	31
SWEETS	Fried pie, apple 1 pie	31
VEGETABLES	Chili con carne w/ beans, cnnd1 cup	31
BREADS	Eng muffin, egg, cheese, bacon1 sandwh	31
SWEETS	Table syrup (corn and maple) 2 tbsp	32
BEVERAGES	Ginger ale 12 fl oz	32
BEVERAGES	Grapejce,frzn,dilutd,swtnd,w/c1 cup	32
FRUITS	Pears, canned, juice pack 1 cup	32
FRUITS	Apples, raw, unpeeled,2 per lb1 apple	32
PASTA	Macaroni, cooked, tender, hot 1 cup	32
PASTA	Spaghetti, cooked, tender 1 cup	32
VEGETABLES	Lima beans,thick seed,frzn,ckd1 cup	32
SWEETS	Gingerbread cake, from mix 1 piece	32
SWEETS	Chocolate chip cookies,refrig 4 cookie	32
VEGETABLES	Potatoes, mashed,frm dehydrted1 cup	32

CHART BY CARBOHYDRATES

	Food	Carbohydrate Grams
DAIRY	Ice cream, vanlla, rich 16% ft1 cup	32
VEGETABLES	Beans,dry,canned,w/frankfurter1 cup	32
BREADS	Pita bread 1 pita	33
DAIRY	Pudding, vanilla, canned 5 oz	33
VEGETABLES	Corn, cooked frm frozn, white 1 cup	34
VEGETABLES	Corn, cooked frm frozn, yellow1 cup	34
BEVERAGES	Pineapple juice, canned,unswtn1 cup	34
VEGETABLES	Potatoes, baked flesh only 1 potato	34
BEVERAGES	Eggnog 1 cup	34
MEATS	Roast beef sandwich 1 sandwh	34
VEGETABLES	Mangos, raw 1 mango	35
FRUITS	Bananas, sliced 1 cup	35
FRUITS	Watermelon, raw 1 piece	35
VEGETABLES	Black-eyed peas, dry, cooked 1 cup	35
VEGETABLES	Lima beans,baby, frzn,cked,drn1 cup	35
VEGETABLES	Potatoes, mashed,recpe,mlk+mar1 cup	35
DAIRY	Nonfat dry milk, instantized 1 cup	35
FRUITS	Apricot nectar, no added vit c1 cup	36
BREADS	Oatmeal w/ raisins cookies 4 cookie	36
SWEETS	Custard pie 1 piece	36
VEGETABLES	Sweetpotatoes, boiled w/o peel1 potato	37
VEGETABLES	Potatoes, mashed,recpe,w/ milk1 cup	37
PASTA	Noodles, egg, cooked 1 cup	37
PASTA	Spaghetti, tom sauce chee,hmrp1 cup	37
SWEETS	Pumpkin pie 1 piece	37
NUTS	Cashew nuts, oil roastd,salted1 cup	37
NUTS	Cashew nuts, oil roastd,unsalt1 cup	37
BEVERAGES	Cranberry juice cocktal w/vitc1 cup	38
FRUITS	Plums, canned, juice pack 1 cup	38
BEVERAGES	Grape juice, canned 1 cup	38
BREADS	Bagels, egg 1 bagel	38
BREADS	Bagels, plain 1 bagel	38
MISCELLANEOUS	Great northn beans,dry,ckd,drn1 cup	38
BREADS	Toaster pastries 1 pastry	38
VEGETABLES	Lentils, dry, cooked 1 cup	38
DAIRY	Ice milk, vanilla,softserv 3% 1 cup	38
BREADS	Coffeecake, crumb, from mix 1 piece	38
DAIRY	Ice cream, vanlla, soft serve 1 cup	38
MEATS	Hamburger, 4oz patty 1 sandwh	38
BEVERAGES	Grapefruit, canned, syrup pack1 cup	39
FRUITS	Pineapple, canned, juice pack 1 cup	39
BEVERAGES	Lemon-lime soda 12 fl oz	39

CHART BY CARBOHYDRATES

	Food	Carbohydrate Grams
PASTA	Spaghetti, tom sauce chees,cnd1 cup	39
SWEETS	Yellowcake w/ chocfrstng,comml1 piece	39
BREADS	Pizza, cheese 1 slice	39
PASTA	Spaghetti,meatballs,tomsa,hmrp1 cup	39
FISH	Fish sandwich, reg, w/ cheese 1 sandwh	39
MEATS	Beef potpie, home recipe 1 piece	39
RICE	Rice, white, instant, cooked 1 cup	40
VEGETABLES	Blackeye peas,immtr,frzn,cked 1 cup	40
VEGETABLES	Pea beans, dry, cooked,drained1 cup	40
SWEETS	Devil's food cake,chocfrst,fmx1 piece	40
SWEETS	Yellow cake w/ choc frst,frmix1 piece	40
BREADS	Bread stuffing,from mx,moist 1 cup	40
PASTA	Macaroni and cheese, home rcpe1 cup	40
MEATS	Cheeseburger, 4oz patty 1 sandwh	40
FRUITS	Tangerines, canned, light syrp1 cup	41
BEVERAGES	Cola, regular 12 fl oz	41
BEVERAGES	Pepper-type soda 12 fl oz	41
VEGETABLES	Corn,cnnd,whl krnl,whte,no sal1 cup	41
VEGETABLES	Corn,cnnd,whl krnl,whte,w/salt1 cup	41
VEGETABLES	Corn,cnnd,whl krnl,yllw,no sal1 cup	41
VEGETABLES	Corn,cnnd,whl krnl,yllw,w/salt1 cup	41
RICE	Rice, white, parboiled, cooked1 cup	41
VEGETABLES	Black beans, dry, cooked,drand1 cup	41
FISH	Fish sandwich, lge, w/o cheese1 sandwh	41
FRUITS	Apples, dried, sulfured 10 rings	42
BEVERAGES	Root beer 12 fl oz	42
SWEETS	Fig bars 4 cookie	42
VEGETABLES	Peas, split, dry, cooked 1 cup	42
VEGETABLES	Red kidney beans, dry, canned 1 cup	42
SWEETS	White cake w/ wht frstng,comml1 piece	42
POULTRY	Chicken potpie, home recipe 1 piece	42
DAIRY	Yogurt, w/ lofat milk,fruitflv8 oz	43
VEGETABLES	Potatoes, hashed brown,fr frzn1 cup	44
SWEETS	Coconut, dried, sweetnd,shredd1 cup	44
FRUITS	Prune juice, canned 1 cup	45
VEGETABLES	Chickpeas, cooked, drained 1 cup	45
NUTS	Cashew nuts, dry roastd,unsalt1 cup	45
NUTS	Cashew nuts, dry roasted,saltd1 cup	45
BEVERAGES	Grape soda 12 fl oz	46
VEGETABLES	Orange soda 12 fl oz	46
VEGETABLES	Corn, cnnd,crm stl,whit,no sal1 cup	46
VEGETABLES	Corn, cnnd,crm stl,whit,w/salt1 cup	46

CHART BY CARBOHYDRATES

	Food		Carbohydrate Grams
DAIRY	Nonfat dry milk, instantized	1 envlpe	47
FRUITS	Plantains, cooked	1 cup	48
FRUITS	Fruit cocktail,cnnd,heavysyrup	1 cup	48
BREADS	Pretzels, twisted, thin	10 pretz	48
VEGETABLES	Beans,dry,canned,w/pork+tomsce	1 cup	48
SWEETS	Sheetcake,w/o frstng,homerecip	1 piece	48
SWEETS	Carrot cake,cremchese frst,rec	1 piece	48
FRUITS	Pears, canned, heavy syrup	1 cup	49
SAUCES	Tomato paste, canned w/o salt	1 cup	49
SAUCES	Tomato paste, canned with salt	1 cup	49
VEGETABLES	Lima beans, dry, cooked,draned	1 cup	49
VEGETABLES	Pinto beans,dry,cooked,drained	1 cup	49
FRUITS	Blueberries, frozen, sweetened	1 cup	50
RICE	Rice, white, cooked	1 cup	50
RICE	Rice, brown, cooked	1 cup	50
DAIRY	Shakes, thick, vanilla	10 oz	50
BREADS	Bread stuffing,from mx,drytype	1 cup	50
FRUITS	Peaches, canned, heavy syrup	1 cup	51
FRUITS	Applesauce, canned, sweetened	1 cup	51
FRUITS	Peaches, dried,cooked,unswetnd	1 cup	51
VEGETABLES	Potatoes, baked with skin	1 potato	51
VEGETABLES	Refried beans, canned	1 cup	51
FRUITS	Pineapple, canned, heavy syrup	1 cup	52
SWEETS	Lemon meringue pie	1 piece	53
VEGETABLES	Beans,dry,canned,w/pork+swtsce	1 cup	54
FRUITS	Apricots, dried, cooked,unswtn	1 cup	55
FRUITS	Apricot, canned, heavy syrup	1 cup	55
SWEETS	Blueberry pie	1 piece	55
FRUITS	Plantains, raw	1 plantn	57
VEGETABLES	Sweetpotatoes, canned, mashed	1 cup	59
SWEETS	Sherbet, 2% fat	1 cup	59
SWEETS	Creme pie	1 piece	59
DAIRY	Buttermilk, dried	1 cup	59
FRUITS	Prunes, dried, cooked,unswtned	1 cup	60
FRUITS	Plums, canned, heavy syrup	1 cup	60
FRUITS	Peaches, frozen,swetned,w/vitc	1 cup	60
DAIRY	Shakes, thick, chocolate	10 oz	60
SWEETS	Peach pie	1 piece	60
SWEETS	Apple pie	1 piece	60
NUTS	Dates	10 dates	61
SWEETS	Cherry pie	1 piece	61
FRUITS	Blueberries, frozen, sweetened	10 oz	62

CHART BY CARBOHYDRATES

	Food		Carbohydrate Grams
FRUITS	Peaches, frozen,swetned,w/vitc	10 oz	68
SAUCES	Catsup	1 cup	69
SWEETS	Pecan pie	1 piece	71
BEVERAGES	Grapefrt jce,frzn,cncn,unswten	6 fl oz	72
BREADS	Rolls, hoagie or submarine	1 roll	72
BREADS	Breadcrumbs, dry, grated	1 cup	73
FRUITS	Strawberries, frozen, sweetend	10 oz	74
FRUITS	Raspberries, frozen, sweetened	10 oz	74
FRUITS	Rhubarb, cooked, added sugar	1 cup	75
MISCELLANEOUS	Cake or pastry flour, sifted	1 cup	76
NUTS	Chestnuts, european, roasted	1 cup	76
SWEETS	Sheetcake,w/ whfrstng,homercip	1 piece	77
MISCELLANEOUS	Buckwheat flour, light, sifted	1 cup	78
BREADS	Piecrust,from home recipe	1 shell	79
FRUITS	Apricots, dried, uncooked	1 cup	80
BEVERAGES	Orange juice,frozen concentrte	6 fl oz	81
SWEETS	Whole-wheat flour,hrd wht,stir	1 cup	85
BREADS	Wheat flour, all-purpose,siftd	1 cup	88
BREADS	Cornmeal,whole-grnd,unbolt,dry	1 cup	90
BREADS	Cornmeal,bolted,dry form	1 cup	91
BREADS	Self-rising flour, unsifted	1 cup	93
BREADS	Wheat flour, all-purpose,unsif	1 cup	95
BEVERAGES	Grapejce,frzn,concen,swtnd,w/c	6 fl oz	96
SWEETS	Semisweet chocolate	1 cup	97
FRUITS	Peaches, dried	1 cup	98
SWEETS	Sugar, powdered, sifted	1 cup	100
BEVERAGES	Limeade,concentrate,frzn,undil	6 fl oz	108
FRUITS	Cranberry sauce, canned,swtnd	1 cup	108
BREADS	Cornmeal,degermed,enriched,dry	1 cup	108
BEVERAGES	Lemonade,concentrate,frz,undil	6 fl oz	112
FRUITS	Raisins	1 cup	115
FRUITS	Figs, dried	10 figs	122
MISCELLANEOUS	Carob flour	1 cup	126
PASTA	Bulgur, uncooked	1 cup	129
NUTS	Dates, chopped	1 cup	131
BREADS	Piecrust, from mix	2 crust	141
RICE	Rice, white, raw	1 cup	149
RICE	Rice, white, parboiled, raw	1 cup	150
BREADS	Danish pastry, plain, no nuts	1 ring	152
VEGETABLES	Barley, pearled,light, uncookd	1 cup	158
SWEETS	Sweetened condensed milk cnnd	1 cup	166
SWEETS	Sugar, white, granulated	1 cup	199

CHART BY CARBOHYDRATES

	Food		Carbohydrate Grams
BREADS	Oatmeal bread	1 loaf	212
BREADS	Mixed grain bread	1 loaf	212
BREADS	Wheat bread	1 loaf	213
SWEETS	Custard pie	1 pie	213
BREADS	Pumpernickel bread	1 loaf	218
BREADS	Rye bread, light	1 loaf	218
BREADS	White bread	1 loaf	222
SWEETS	Pumpkin pie	1 pie	223
BREADS	Coffeecake, crumb, from mix	1 cake	225
BREADS	Cracked-wheat bread	1 loaf	227
BREADS	French or vienna bread	1 loaf	230
DAIRY	Ice milk, vanilla, 4% fat	1/2 gal	232
BREADS	Raisin bread	1 loaf	239
DAIRY	Ice cream, vanlla, regulr 11%	1/2 galn	254
BREADS	Italian bread	1 loaf	256
DAIRY	Ice cream, vanlla, rich 16% ft	1/2 gal	256
SWEETS	Pound cake, commercial	1 loaf	257
SWEETS	Pound cake, from home recipe	1 loaf	265
SWEETS	Honey	1 cup	279
SWEETS	Gingerbread cake, from mix	1 cake	291
SWEETS	Lemon meringue pie	1 pie	317
SWEETS	Cheesecake	1 cake	317
SWEETS	Blueberry pie	1 pie	330
SWEETS	Angelfood cake, from mix	1 cake	342
SWEETS	Creme pie	1 pie	351
SWEETS	Apple pie	1 pie	360
SWEETS	Peach pie	1 pie	361
SWEETS	Cherry pie	1 pie	363
SWEETS	Pecan pie	1 pie	423
SWEETS	Sheetcake w/o frstng,homerecip	1 cake	434
SWEETS	Sherbet, 2% fat	1/2 gal	469
SWEETS	Yellowcake w/ chocfrstng,comml	1 cake	620
SWEETS	Yellow cake w/ choc frst,frmix	1 cake	638
SWEETS	Devil's food cake,chocfrst,fmx	1 cake	645
SWEETS	White cake w/ wht frstng,comml	1 cake	670
SWEETS	Sheetcake,w/ whfrstng,homercip	1 cake	694
SWEETS	Carrot cake,cremchese frst,rec	1 cake	775
SWEETS	Fruitcake,dark, from homerecip	1 cake	783

CHART BY FAT GRAMS

CHART BY FAT GRAMS

	Food	Fat Grams
VEGETABLES	Alfalfa seeds, sprouted, raw 1 cup	0
SWEETS	Angelfood cake, from mix 1 piece	0
BEVERAGES	Apple juice, canned 1 cup	0
FRUITS	Apples, dried, sulfured 10 rings	0
FRUITS	Apples, raw, peeled, sliced 1 cup	0
FRUITS	Apples, raw, unpeeled,3 per lb1 apple	0
FRUITS	Applesauce, canned, sweetened 1 cup	0
FRUITS	Applesauce, canned,unsweetened1 cup	0
FRUITS	Apricot nectar, no added vit c1 cup	0
FRUITS	Apricot, canned, heavy syrup 1 cup	0
FRUITS	Apricot, canned, heavy syrup 3 halves	0
FRUITS	Apricots, canned, juice pack 1 cup	0
FRUITS	Apricots, canned, juice pack 3 halves	0
FRUITS	Apricots, dried, cooked,unswtn1 cup	0
FRUITS	Apricots, raw 3 aprcot	0
VEGETABLES	Artichokes, globe, cooked, drn1 artchk	0
VEGETABLES	Asparagus, ckd frm frz,dr,sper4 spears	0
VEGETABLES	Asparagus, ckd frm raw,dr,sper4 spears	0
VEGETABLES	Asparagus,canned,spears,nosalt4 spears	0
VEGETABLES	Asparagus,canned,spears,w/salt4 spears	0
MISCELLANEOUS	Baking powder, low sodium 1 tsp	0
MISCELLANEOUS	Baking powder, strght phosphat1 tsp	0
MISCELLANEOUS	Baking powder,sas, ca po4 1 tsp	0
BREADS	Baking powder,sas,capo4+caso4 1 tsp	0
SAUCES	Barbecue sauce 1 tbsp	0
VEGETABLES	Bean sprouts, mung, cookd,dran1 cup	0
VEGETABLES	Bean sprouts, mung, raw 1 cup	0
BEVERAGES	Beer, light 12 fl oz	0
BEVERAGES	Beer, regular 12 fl oz	0
VEGETABLES	Beet greens, cooked, drained 1 cup	0
VEGETABLES	Beets, canned, drained,no salt1 cup	0
VEGETABLES	Beets, canned, drained,w/ salt1 cup	0
VEGETABLES	Beets, cooked, drained, diced 1 cup	0
VEGETABLES	Beets, cooked, drained, whole 2 beets	0
FRUITS	Blueberries, frozen, sweetened1 cup	0
FRUITS	Blueberries, frozen, sweetened10 oz	0
CEREAL	Bran flakes, post 1 oz	0

CHART BY FAT GRAMS

	Food	Fat Grams
VEGETABLES	Broccoli, frzn, cooked, draned1 cup	0
VEGETABLES	Broccoli, frzn, cooked, draned1 piece	0
VEGETABLES	Broccoli, raw, cooked, drained1 cup	0
VEGETABLES	Cabbage, chinese, pak-choi,ckd1 cup	0
VEGETABLES	Cabbage, chinese,pe-tsai, raw 1 cup	0
VEGETABLES	Cabbage, common, cooked, drned1 cup	0
VEGETABLES	Cabbage, common, raw 1 cup	0
VEGETABLES	Cabbage, red, raw 1 cup	0
VEGETABLES	Cabbage, savoy, raw 1 cup	0
MISCELLANEOUS	Carob flour 1 cup	0
VEGETABLES	Carrots, canned, drn, w/ salt 1 cup	0
VEGETABLES	Carrots, canned,drnd, w/o salt1 cup	0
VEGETABLES	Carrots, cooked from frozen 1 cup	0
VEGETABLES	Carrots, cooked from raw 1 cup	0
VEGETABLES	Carrots, raw, grated 1 cup	0
VEGETABLES	Carrots, raw, whole 1 carrot	0
SAUCES	Catsup 1 tbsp	0
VEGETABLES	Cauliflower, cooked from frozn1 cup	0
VEGETABLES	Cauliflower, cooked from raw 1 cup	0
VEGETABLES	Cauliflower, raw 1 cup	0
VEGETABLES	Celery, pascal type, raw,piece1 cup	0
VEGETABLES	Celery, pascal type, raw,stalk1 stalk	0
FRUITS	Cherries, sour,red,cannd,water1 cup	0
POULTRY	Chicken chow mein, canned 1 cup	0
SPICES	Chili powder 1 tsp	0
SPICES	Cinnamon 1 tsp	0
BEVERAGES	Club soda 12 fl oz	0
BEVERAGES	Coffee, brewed 6 fl oz	0
BEVERAGES	Coffee, instant, prepared 6 fl oz	0
BEVERAGES	Cola, diet, aspartame only 12 fl oz	0
BEVERAGES	Cola, diet, asprtame + sacchrn12 fl oz	0
BEVERAGES	Cola, diet, saccharin only 12 fl oz	0
BEVERAGES	Cola, regular 12 fl oz	0
VEGETABLES	Collards, cooked from raw 1 cup	0
CEREAL	Corn flakes, kellogg's 1 oz	0
CEREAL	Corn flakes, toasties 1 oz	0
BREADS	Corn grits, cooked, instant 1 pkt	0
BREADS	Corn grits,ckd,reg,whte,nosalt1 cup	0
BREADS	Corn grits,ckd,reg,whte,w/salt1 cup	0
BREADS	Corn grits,ckd,reg,yllw,nosalt1 cup	0
BREADS	Corn grits,ckd,reg,yllw,w/salt1 cup	0

CHART BY FAT GRAMS

	Food	Fat Grams
VEGETABLES	Corn, cooked frm frozn, white 1 cup	0
VEGETABLES	Corn, cooked frm frozn, white 1 ear	0
VEGETABLES	Corn, cooked frm frozn, yellow1 cup	0
VEGETABLES	Corn, cooked frm frozn, yellow1 ear	0
BREADS	Cornmeal,degermed,enrched,cook1 cup	0
BEVERAGES	Cranberry juice cocktal w/vitc1 cup	0
FRUITS	Cranberry sauce, canned,swtnd 1 cup	0
DAIRY	Cream of wheat,ckd,mix n eat 1 pkt	0
DAIRY	Crm wheat,ckd, quick, no salt 1 cup	0
DAIRY	Crm wheat,ckd,quick, w/ salt 1 cup	0
DAIRY	Crm wheat,ckd,reg,inst,no salt1 cup	0
DAIRY	Crm wheat,ckd,reg,inst,w/salt 1 cup	0
VEGETABLES	Cucumber, w/ peel 6 slices	0
SPICES	Curry powder 1 tsp	0
NUTS	Dates 10 dates	0
VEGETABLES	Eggplant, cooked, steamed 1 cup	0
DAIRY	Eggs, raw, white 1 white	0
VEGETABLES	Endive, curly, raw 1 cup	0
FRUITS	Fruit cocktail,cnnd,heavysyrup1 cup	0
FRUITS	Fruit cocktail,cnnd,juice pack1 cup	0
BEVERAGES	Fruit punch drink, canned 6 fl oz	0
SPICES	Garlic powder 1 tsp	0
MISCELLANEOUS	Gelatin dessert, prepared 1/2 cup	0
MISCELLANEOUS	Gelatin, dry 1 envelp	0
BEVERAGES	Gin,rum,vodka,whisky 80-proof 1.5 f oz	0
BEVERAGES	Gin,rum,vodka,whisky 86-proof 1.5 f oz	0
BEVERAGES	Gin,rum,vodka,whisky 90-proof 1.5 f oz	0
BEVERAGES	Ginger ale 12 fl oz	0
BEVERAGES	Grape drink, canned 6 fl oz	0
BEVERAGES	Grape juice, canned 1 cup	0
BEVERAGES	Grape soda 12 fl oz	0
BEVERAGES	Grapefrt jce,frzn,dltd,unswten1 cup	0
BEVERAGES	Grapefruit juice, canned,swtnd1 cup	0
BEVERAGES	Grapefruit juice, canned,unswt1 cup	0
BEVERAGES	Grapefruit juice, raw 1 cup	0
BEVERAGES	Grapefruit, canned, syrup pack1 cup	0
BEVERAGES	Grapefruit, raw, pink 1/2 frut	0
BEVERAGES	Grapefruit, raw, white 1/2 frut	0
BEVERAGES	Grapejce,frzn,dilutd,swtnd,w/c1 cup	0
CEREAL	Grape-nuts cereal 1 oz	0
FRUITS	Grapes, european, raw, thompsn10 grape	0

CHART BY FAT GRAMS

	Food	Fat Grams
FRUITS	Grapes, european, raw, tokay 10 grape	0
SWEETS	Gum drops	1 oz	0
SWEETS	Hard candy	1 oz	0
SWEETS	Honey	1 cup	0
SWEETS	Honey	1 tbsp	0
FRUITS	Honeydew melon, raw	1/10 mel	0
DAIRY	Imitatn whipd toping,pwdrd,prp1 tbsp	0
BREADS	Italian bread	1 slice	0
SAUCES	Italian salad dressing,localor1 tbsp	0
FRUITS	Jams and preserves	1 pkt	0
FRUITS	Jams and preserves	1 tbsp	0
FRUITS	Jellies	1 pkt	0
FRUITS	Jellies	1 tbsp	0
SWEETS	Jelly beans	1 oz	0
VEGETABLES	Jerusalem-artichoke, raw	1 cup	0
FRUITS	Kiwifruit, raw	1 kiwi	0
FRUITS	Lemon juice, canned	1 tbsp	0
FRUITS	Lemon juice, raw	1 cup	0
BEVERAGES	Lemonade,concen,frzen,diluted 6 fl oz	0
BEVERAGES	Lemonade,concentrate,frz,undil6 fl oz	0
BEVERAGES	Lemon-lime soda	12 fl oz	0
FRUITS	Lemons, raw	1 lemon	0
VEGETABLES	Lettuce, butterhead, raw,head 1 head	0
VEGETABLES	Lettuce, butterhead, raw,leave1 leaf	0
VEGETABLES	Lettuce, crisphead, raw,pieces1 cup	0
VEGETABLES	Lettuce, crisphead, raw,wedge 1 wedge	0
VEGETABLES	Lettuce, looseleaf	1 cup	0
FRUITS	Lime juice, raw	1 cup	0
BEVERAGES	Limeade,concen,frozen,diluted 6 fl oz	0
BEVERAGES	Limeade,concentrate,frzn,undil6 fl oz	0
PASTA	Macaroni, cooked, tender,cold 1 cup	0
SWEETS	Marshmallows	1 oz	0
BREADS	Melba toast, plain	1 piece	0
DAIRY	Milk, skim, no added milksolid1 cup	0
SWEETS	Molasses, cane, blackstrap	2 tbsp	0
VEGETABLES	Mushrooms, canned, drnd,w/salt1 cup	0
VEGETABLES	Mushrooms, raw	1 cup	0
VEGETABLES	Mustard greens, cooked, draned1 cup	0
SAUCES	Mustard, prepared, yellow	1 tsp	0
DAIRY	Nonfat dry milk, instantized	1 cup	0
VEGETABLES	Okra pods, cooked	8 pods	0

CHART BY FAT GRAMS

	Food		Fat Grams
SPICES	Onion powder	1 tsp	0
SOUPS	Onion soup, dehydratd, prepred	1 pkt	0
SOUPS	Onion soup, dehydrtd, unprpred	1 pkt	0
VEGETABLES	Onions, raw, chopped	1 cup	0
VEGETABLES	Onions, raw, cooked, drained	1 cup	0
VEGETABLES	Onions, raw, sliced	1 cup	0
VEGETABLES	Onions, spring, raw	6 onion	0
BEVERAGES	Orange + grapefruit juce,cannd	1 cup	0
BEVERAGES	Orange juice, canned	1 cup	0
BEVERAGES	Orange juice, raw	1 cup	0
BEVERAGES	Orange juice,frozen concentrte	6 fl oz	0
BEVERAGES	Orange juice,frzn,cncn,diluted	1 cup	0
BEVERAGES	Orange soda	12 fl oz	0
FRUITS	Oranges, raw	1 orange	0
FRUITS	Oranges, raw, sections	1 cup	0
SPICES	Oregano	1 tsp	0
FRUITS	Papayas, raw	1 cup	0
SPICES	Paprika	1 tsp	0
SPICES	Parsley, freeze-dried	1 tbsp	0
VEGETABLES	Parsley, raw	10 sprig	0
VEGETABLES	Parsnips, cooked, drained	1 cup	0
FRUITS	Peaches, canned, heavy syrup	1 cup	0
FRUITS	Peaches, canned, heavy syrup	1 half	0
FRUITS	Peaches, canned, juice pack	1 cup	0
FRUITS	Peaches, canned, juice pack	1 half	0
FRUITS	Peaches, frozen,swetned,w/vitc	1 cup	0
FRUITS	Peaches, frozen,swetned,w/vitc	10 oz	0
FRUITS	Peaches, raw	1 peach	0
FRUITS	Peaches, raw, sliced	1 cup	0
FRUITS	Pears, canned, heavy syrup	1 cup	0
FRUITS	Pears, canned, heavy syrup	1 half	0
FRUITS	Pears, canned, juice pack	1 cup	0
FRUITS	Pears, canned, juice pack	1 half	0
VEGETABLES	Peas, edible pod, cooked,drned	1 cup	0
VEGETABLES	Peas,grn, frozen cooked,draned	1 cup	0
SPICES	Pepper, black	1 tsp	0
VEGETABLES	Peppers, hot chili, raw, green	1 pepper	0
VEGETABLES	Peppers, hot chili, raw, red	1 pepper	0
VEGETABLES	Peppers, sweet, cooked, green	1 pepper	0
VEGETABLES	Peppers, sweet, cooked, red	1 pepper	0
VEGETABLES	Peppers, sweet, raw, green	1 pepper	0

CHART BY FAT GRAMS

	Food	Fat Grams
VEGETABLES	Peppers, sweet, raw, red 1 pepper	0
BEVERAGES	Pepper-type soda 12 fl oz	0
VEGETABLES	Pickles, cucumber, dill 1 pickle	0
VEGETABLES	Pickles, cucumber, fresh pack 2 slices	0
VEGETABLES	Pickles, cucumber, swt gherkin 1 pickle	0
BEVERAGES	Pineapple juice, canned, unswtn 1 cup	0
FRUITS	Pineapple, canned, heavy syrup 1 cup	0
FRUITS	Pineapple, canned, heavy syrup 1 slice	0
FRUITS	Pineapple, canned, juice pack 1 cup	0
FRUITS	Pineapple, canned, juice pack 1 slice	0
BEVERAGES	Pineapple-grapefruit juicedrnk 6 fl oz	0
FRUITS	Plantains, cooked 1 cup	0
FRUITS	Plums, canned, heavy syrup 1 cup	0
FRUITS	Plums, canned, heavy syrup 3 plums	0
FRUITS	Plums, canned, juice pack 1 cup	0
FRUITS	Plums, canned, juice pack 3 plums	0
FRUITS	Plums, raw, 1-1/2-in diam 1 plum	0
FRUITS	Plums, raw, 2-1/8-in diam 1 plum	0
NUTS	Popcorn, air-popped, unsalted 1 cup	0
SWEETS	Popsicle 1 popcle	0
VEGETABLES	Potatoes, baked flesh only 1 potato	0
VEGETABLES	Potatoes, baked with skin 1 potato	0
VEGETABLES	Potatoes, boiled, peeled after 1 potato	0
VEGETABLES	Potatoes, boiled, peeled befor 1 potato	0
BREADS	Pretzels, stick 10 pretz	0
CEREAL	Product 19 cereal 1 oz	0
FRUITS	Prune juice, canned 1 cup	0
FRUITS	Prunes, dried 5 large	0
FRUITS	Prunes, dried, cooked, unswtned 1 cup	0
VEGETABLES	Pumpkin, cooked from raw 1 cup	0
VEGETABLES	Radishes, raw 4 radish	0
FRUITS	Raisins 1 packet	0
FRUITS	Raspberries, frozen, sweetened 1 cup	0
FRUITS	Raspberries, frozen, sweetened 10 oz	0
SAUCES	Relish, sweet 1 tbsp	0
FRUITS	Rhubarb, cooked, added sugar 1 cup	0
BREADS	Rice krispies cereal 1 oz	0
RICE	Rice, white, cooked 1 cup	0
RICE	Rice, white, instant, cooked 1 cup	0
RICE	Rice, white, parboiled, cooked 1 cup	0
BEVERAGES	Root beer 12 fl oz	0

CHART BY FAT GRAMS

Food			Fat Grams
SPICES	Salt	1 tsp	0
VEGETABLES	Sauerkraut, canned	1 cup	0
VEGETABLES	Seaweed, kelp, raw	1 oz	0
VEGETABLES	Snap bean,cnnd,drnd,green,salt	1 cup	0
VEGETABLES	Snap bean,cnnd,drnd,grn,nosalt	1 cup	0
VEGETABLES	Snap bean,cnnd,drnd,yllw, salt	1 cup	0
VEGETABLES	Snap bean,cnnd,drnd,yllw,nosal	1 cup	0
VEGETABLES	Snap bean,frz,ckd,drnd,green	1 cup	0
VEGETABLES	Snap bean,frz,ckd,drnd,yellow	1 cup	0
VEGETABLES	Snap bean,raw,ckd,drnd,green	1 cup	0
VEGETABLES	Snap bean,raw,ckd,drnd,yellow	1 cup	0
SAUCES	Soy sauce	1 tbsp	0
CEREAL	Special K cereal	1 oz	0
VEGETABLES	Spinach, cooked fr frzen, drnd	1 cup	0
VEGETABLES	Spinach, cooked from raw, drnd	1 cup	0
VEGETABLES	Spinach, raw	1 cup	0
FRUITS	Strawberries, frozen, sweetend	1 cup	0
FRUITS	Strawberries, frozen, sweetend	10 oz	0
CEREAL	Sugar frosted flakes, kellogg	1 oz	0
SWEETS	Sugar, brown, pressed down	1 cup	0
SWEETS	Sugar, powdered, sifted	1 cup	0
SWEETS	Sugar, white, granulated	1 cup	0
SWEETS	Sugar, white, granulated	1 pkt	0
SWEETS	Sugar, white, granulated	1 tbsp	0
CEREAL	Super sugar crisp cereal	1 oz	0
VEGETABLES	Sweetpotatoes, baked, peeled	1 potato	0
VEGETABLES	Sweetpotatoes, boiled w/o peel	1 potato	0
VEGETABLES	Sweetpotatoes, cnned, vac pack	1 piece	0
SWEETS	Syrup, chocolate flavored thin	2 tbsp	0
SWEETS	Table syrup (corn and maple)	2 tbsp	0
FRUITS	Tangerine juice, canned,swtned	1 cup	0
FRUITS	Tangerines, canned, light syrp	1 cup	0
FRUITS	Tangerines, raw	1 tangrn	0
BEVERAGES	Tea, brewed	8 fl oz	0
BEVERAGES	Tea, instant,preprd,unsweetend	8 fl oz	0
BEVERAGES	Tea,instant,prepard,sweetened	8 fl oz	0
BEVERAGES	Tomato juice, canned w/o salt	1 cup	0
BEVERAGES	Tomato juice, canned with salt	1 cup	0
SAUCES	Tomato puree, canned w/o salt	1 cup	0
SAUCES	Tomato puree, canned with salt	1 cup	0
SAUCES	Tomato sauce, canned with salt	1 cup	0

CHART BY FAT GRAMS

	Food		Fat Grams
VEGETABLES	Tomatoes, raw	1 tomato	0
CEREAL	Trix cereal	1 oz	0
VEGETABLES	Turnip greens, cooked from raw	1 cup	0
VEGETABLES	Turnips, cooked, diced	1 cup	0
BEVERAGES	Vegetable juice cocktail, cnnd	1 cup	0
VEGETABLES	Vegetables, mixed, canned	1 cup	0
VEGETABLES	Vegetables, mixed, cked fr frz	1 cup	0
SAUCES	Vinegar, cider	1 tbsp	0
NUTS	Water chestnuts, canned	1 cup	0
CEREAL	Wheaties cereal	1 oz	0
BEVERAGES	Wine, dessert	3.5 f oz	0
BEVERAGES	Wine, table, red	3.5 f oz	0
BEVERAGES	Wine, table, white	3.5 f oz	0
MISCELLANEOUS	Yeast, bakers, dry, active	1 pkg	0
MISCELLANEOUS	Yeast, brewers, dry	1 tbsp	0
DAIRY	Yogurt, w/ nonfat milk	8 oz	0
CEREAL	All-bran cereal	1 oz	1
FRUITS	Apples, raw, unpeeled,2 per lb	1 apple	1
FRUITS	Apricots, dried, uncooked	1 cup	1
VEGETABLES	Asparagus, ckd frm frz,drn,cut	1 cup	1
VEGETABLES	Asparagus, ckd frm raw, dr,cut	1 cup	1
VEGETABLES	Bamboo shoots, canned, drained	1 cup	1
FRUITS	Bananas	1 banana	1
FRUITS	Bananas, sliced	1 cup	1
SOUPS	Beef broth, boulln, consm,cnnd	1 cup	1
VEGETABLES	Black beans, dry, cooked,drand	1 cup	1
FRUITS	Blackberries, raw	1 cup	1
VEGETABLES	Blackeye peas, immatr,raw,cked	1 cup	1
VEGETABLES	Blackeye peas,immtr,frzn,cked	1 cup	1
VEGETABLES	Black-eyed peas, dry, cooked	1 cup	1
FRUITS	Blueberries, raw	1 cup	1
BREADS	Boston brown bread,w/whtecrnm	1 slice	1
BREADS	Boston brown bread,w/yllwcrnml	1 slice	1
SOUPS	Bouillon, dehydrtd, unprepared	1 pkt	1
CEREAL	Bran flakes, kellogg's	1 oz	1
VEGETABLES	Broccoli, raw	1 spear	1
VEGETABLES	Broccoli, raw, cooked, drained	1 spear	1
VEGETABLES	Brussels sprouts, frzn, cooked	1 cup	1
VEGETABLES	Brussels sprouts, raw, cooked	1 cup	1
MISCELLANEOUS	Buckwheat flour, light, sifted	1 cup	1
MISCELLANEOUS	Cake or pastry flour, sifted	1 cup	1

CHART BY FAT GRAMS

	Food		Fat Grams
FRUITS	Cantaloup, raw	1/2 meln	1
SAUCES	Catsup	1 cup	1
SPICES	Celery seed	1 tsp	1
FRUITS	Cherries, sweet, raw	10 chery	1
POULTRY	Chicken liver, cooked	1 liver	1
SOUPS	Chicken noodle soup,dehyd,prpd	1 pkt	1
FISH	Clams, raw	3 oz	1
SWEETS	Coca pwdr w/o nonfat dry milk	3/4 oz	1
SWEETS	Cocoa pwdr w/ nofat drmlk,prpd	1 servng	1
SWEETS	Cocoa pwdr with nonfat drymilk	1 oz	1
VEGETABLES	Collards, cooked from frozen	1 cup	1
VEGETABLES	Corn, cnnd,crm stl,whit,no sal	1 cup	1
VEGETABLES	Corn, cnnd,crm stl,whit,w/salt	1 cup	1
VEGETABLES	Corn, cnnd,crm stl,yllw,no sal	1 cup	1
VEGETABLES	Corn, cnnd,crm stl,yllw,w/salt	1 cup	1
VEGETABLES	Corn, cooked from raw, white	1 ear	1
VEGETABLES	Corn, cooked from raw, yellow	1 ear	1
VEGETABLES	Corn,cnnd,whl krnl,whte,no sal	1 cup	1
VEGETABLES	Corn,cnnd,whl krnl,whte,w/salt	1 cup	1
VEGETABLES	Corn,cnnd,whl krnl,yllw,no sal	1 cup	1
VEGETABLES	Corn,cnnd,whl krnl,yllw,w/salt	1 cup	1
DAIRY	Cottage cheese,uncreamed	1 cup	1
BREADS	Cracked-wheat bread	1 slice	1
BREADS	Cracked-wheat bread, toasted	1 slice	1
VEGETABLES	Dandelion greens, cooked, drnd	1 cup	1
NUTS	Dates, chopped	1 cup	1
BREADS	English muffins, plain	1 muffin	1
BREADS	English muffins, plain, toastd	1 muffin	1
BEVERAGES	Evaporated milk, skim, canned	1 cup	1
FISH	Flounder or sole, baked,w/ofat	3 oz	1
BREADS	French bread	1 slice	1
CEREAL	Froot loops cereal	1 oz	1
CEREAL	Golden grahams cereal	1 oz	1
SWEETS	Graham cracker, plain	2 crackr	1
BEVERAGES	Grapefrt jce,frzn,cncn,unswten	6 fl oz	1
BEVERAGES	Grapejce,frzn,concen,swtnd,w/c	6 fl oz	1
MISCELLANEOUS	Great northn beans,dry,ckd,drn	1 cup	1
CEREAL	Honey nut cheerios cereal	1 oz	1
DAIRY	Imitation creamers, liquid frz	1 tbsp	1
DAIRY	Imitation creamers, powdered	1 tsp	1
DAIRY	Imitation whipped topping,frzn	1 tbsp	1

CHART BY FAT GRAMS

Food		Fat Grams
	Food	Fat Grams
DAIRY	Imitatn whipd toping,pressrzd 1 tbsp	1
VEGETABLES	Kale, cooked from frozen 1 cup	1
VEGETABLES	Kale, cooked from raw 1 cup	1
FRUITS	Lemon juice, canned 1 cup	1
BEVERAGES	Lemon juice,frzn,single-strngh6 fl oz	1
VEGETABLES	Lentils, dry, cooked 1 cup	1
VEGETABLES	Lettuce, crisphead, raw, head 1 head	1
VEGETABLES	Lima beans, dry, cooked,draned1 cup	1
VEGETABLES	Lima beans,baby, frzn,cked,drn1 cup	1
VEGETABLES	Lima beans,thick seed,frzn,ckd1 cup	1
FRUITS	Lime juice,canned 1 cup	1
BREADS	Lucky charms cereal 1 oz	1
PASTA	Macaroni, cooked, firm 1 cup	1
PASTA	Macaroni, cooked, tender, hot 1 cup	1
DAIRY	Malted milk, chocolate, powder3/4 oz	1
VEGETABLES	Mangos, raw 1 mango	1
DAIRY	Milk, skim, added milk solids 1 cup	1
BREADS	Mixed grain bread 1 slice	1
BREADS	Mixed grain bread, toasted 1 slice	1
VEGETABLES	Mushrooms, cooked, drained 1 cup	1
FRUITS	Nectarines, raw 1 nectrn	1
DAIRY	Nonfat dry milk, instantized 1 envlpe	1
BREADS	Oatmeal bread 1 slice	1
BREADS	Oatmeal bread, toasted 1 slice	1
BEVERAGES	Orange juice, chilled 1 cup	1
VEGETABLES	Pea beans, dry, cooked,drained1 cup	1
FRUITS	Peaches, dried 1 cup	1
FRUITS	Peaches, dried,cooked,unswetnd1 cup	1
FRUITS	Pears, raw, bartlett 1 pear	1
FRUITS	Pears, raw, bosc 1 pear	1
FRUITS	Pears, raw, d'anjou 1 pear	1
VEGETABLES	Peas, green,cnnd,drnd, w/ salt1 cup	1
VEGETABLES	Peas, green,cnnd,drnd,w/o salt1 cup	1
VEGETABLES	Peas, split, dry, cooked 1 cup	1
FRUITS	Pineapple, raw, diced 1 cup	1
VEGETABLES	Pinto beans,dry,cooked,drained1 cup	1
BREADS	Pita bread 1 pita	1
FRUITS	Plantains, raw 1 plantn	1
NUTS	Popcorn, sugar syrup coated 1 cup	1
VEGETABLES	Potatoes, mashed,recpe,w/ milk1 cup	1
BREADS	Pretzels, twisted, dutch 1 pretz	1

CHART BY FAT GRAMS

	Food		Fat Grams
BREADS	Pumpernickel bread	1 slice	1
BREADS	Pumpernickel bread, toasted	1 slice	1
VEGETABLES	Pumpkin, canned	1 cup	1
CEREAL	Raisin bran, kellogg's	1 oz	1
CEREAL	Raisin bran, post	1 oz	1
BREADS	Raisin bread	1 slice	1
BREADS	Raisin bread, toasted	1 slice	1
FRUITS	Raisins	1 cup	1
FRUITS	Raspberries, raw	1 cup	1
VEGETABLES	Red kidney beans, dry, canned	1 cup	1
RICE	Rice, brown, cooked	1 cup	1
RICE	Rice, white, parboiled, raw	1 cup	1
RICE	Rice, white, raw	1 cup	1
BREADS	Rye bread, light	1 slice	1
BREADS	Rye bread, light, toasted	1 slice	1
BREADS	Rye wafers, whole-grain	2 wafers	1
BREADS	Saltines	4 crackr	1
BREADS	Self-rising flour, unsifted	1 cup	1
CEREAL	Shredded wheat cereal	1 oz	1
FISH	Shrimp, canned, drained	3 oz	1
BREADS	Snack type crackers	1 crackr	1
PASTA	Spaghetti, cooked, firm	1 cup	1
PASTA	Spaghetti, cooked, tender	1 cup	1
VEGETABLES	Spinach, canned, drnd,w/ salt	1 cup	1
VEGETABLES	Spinach, canned, drnd,w/o salt	1 cup	1
VEGETABLES	Squash, summer, cooked, drain	1 cup	1
VEGETABLES	Squash, winter, baked	1 cup	1
FRUITS	Strawberries, raw	1 cup	1
CEREAL	Sugar smacks cereal	1 oz	1
VEGETABLES	Sweetpotatoes, canned, mashed	1 cup	1
SOUPS	Tomato veg soup, dehyd,prepred	1 pkt	1
VEGETABLES	Tomatoes, canned, s+l, w/ salt	1 cup	1
VEGETABLES	Tomatoes, canned, s+l,w/o salt	1 cup	1
BREADS	Tortillas, corn	1 tortla	1
CEREAL	Total cereal	1 oz	1
FISH	Tuna, cannd, drnd,watr, white	3 oz	1
POULTRY	Turkey loaf, breast meat w/o c	2 slices	1
POULTRY	Turkey loaf, breast meat, w/ c	2 slices	1
VEGETABLES	Turnip greens, cked frm frozen	1 cup	1
BREADS	Vienna bread	1 slice	1
FRUITS	Watermelon, raw, diced	1 cup	1

CHART BY FAT GRAMS

	Food		Fat Grams
BREADS	Wheat bread	1 slice	1
BREADS	Wheat bread, toasted	1 slice	1
BREADS	Wheat flour, all-purpose,siftd	1 cup	1
BREADS	Wheat flour, all-purpose,unsif	1 cup	1
BREADS	Wheat, thin crackers	4 crackr	1
DAIRY	Whipped topping, pressurized	1 tbsp	1
BREADS	White bread cubes	1 cup	1
BREADS	White bread, slice 18 per loaf	1 slice	1
BREADS	White bread, slice 22 per loaf	1 slice	1
BREADS	White bread, toasted 18 per	1 slice	1
BREADS	White bread, toasted 22 per	1 slice	1
SWEETS	Whole-wheat bread	1 slice	1
SWEETS	Whole-wheat bread, toasted	1 slice	1
SAUCES	1000 island, salad drsng,local	1 tbsp	2
SWEETS	Angelfood cake, from mix	1 cake	2
BREADS	Bagels, egg	1 bagel	2
BREADS	Bagels, plain	1 bagel	2
BREADS	Baking pwdr biscuits,refrgdogh	1 biscut	2
VEGETABLES	Barley, pearled,light, uncookd	1 cup	2
SAUCES	Brown gravy from dry mix	1 cup	2
DAIRY	Buttermilk, fluid	1 cup	2
CEREAL	Cheerios cereal	1 oz	2
BREADS	Cheese crackers, sandwch,peant	1 sandwh	2
SAUCES	Chicken gravy from dry mix	1 cup	2
SOUPS	Chicken noodle soup, canned	1 cup	2
SOUPS	Chicken rice soup, canned	1 cup	2
POULTRY	Chicken, roasted, drumstick	1.6 oz	2
SOUPS	Clam chowder, manhattan, cannd	1 cup	2
FISH	Clams, canned, drained	3 oz	2
SAUCES	Cooked salad drssing, home rcp	1 tbsp	2
BREADS	Cornmeal,degermed,enriched,dry	1 cup	2
FRUITS	Figs, dried	10 figs	2
SAUCES	French salad dressing, localor	1 tbsp	2
BEVERAGES	Half and half, cream	1 tbsp	2
DAIRY	Imitatn sour dressing	1 tbsp	2
DAIRY	Malted milk,natural, powder	3/4 oz	2
DAIRY	Milk, lofat, 1%, added solids	1 cup	2
PASTA	Noodles, egg, cooked	1 cup	2
BREADS	Oatmeal,ckd,instnt,flvrd,fortf	1 pkt	2
BREADS	Oatmeal,ckd,instnt,plain,fortf	1 pkt	2
BREADS	Oatmeal,ckd,rg,qck,inst,w/osal	1 cup	2

CHART BY FAT GRAMS

	Food	Fat Grams
BREADS	Oatmeal,ckd,rg,qck,inst,w/salt1 cup	2
VEGETABLES	Olives, canned, green 4 medium	2
VEGETABLES	Olives, canned, ripe, mission 3 small	2
BREADS	Pancakes, buckwheat, from mix 1 pancak	2
BREADS	Pancakes, plain, from mix 1 pancak	2
BREADS	Pancakes, plain, home recipe 1 pancak	2
DAIRY	Parmesan cheese, grated 1 tbsp	2
BREADS	Pretzels, twisted, thin 10 pretz	2
BREADS	Rolls, dinner, commercial 1 roll	2
BREADS	Rolls, frankfurter + hamburger1 roll	2
BREADS	Rolls, hard 1 roll	2
VEGETABLES	Seaweed, spirulina, dried 1 oz	2
PASTA	Spaghetti, tom sauce chees,cnd1 cup	2
SAUCES	Tomato paste, canned w/o salt 1 cup	2
SAUCES	Tomato paste, canned with salt1 cup	2
SOUPS	Tomato soup w/ water, canned 1 cup	2
SOUPS	Vegetable beef soup, canned 1 cup	2
SOUPS	Vegetarian soup, canned 1 cup	2
FRUITS	Watermelon, raw 1 piece	2
BREADS	White bread crumbs, soft 1 cup	2
SWEETS	Whole-wheat flour,hrd wht,stir1 cup	2
SWEETS	Whole-wheat wafers, crackers 2 crackr	2
DAIRY	Yogurt, w/ lofat milk,fruitflv8 oz	2
BREADS	Baking pwdr biscuits,from mix 1 biscut	3
SOUPS	Beef noodle soup, canned 1 cup	3
PASTA	Bulgur, uncooked 1 cup	3
CEREAL	Cap'n crunch cereal 1 oz	3
SWEETS	Caramels, plain or chocolate 1 oz	3
BREADS	Cheese crackers, plain 10 crack	3
NUTS	Chestnuts, european, roasted 1 cup	3
POULTRY	Chicken, roasted, breast 3.0 oz	3
BEVERAGES	Chocolate milk, lowfat 1% 1 cup	3
FISH	Crabmeat, canned 1 cup	3
FISH	Fish sticks, frozen, reheated 1 stick	3
SWEETS	Fudge, chocolate, plain 1 oz	3
DAIRY	Light, coffee or table cream 1 tbsp	3
DAIRY	Margarine, spread,hard,60% fat1 pat	3
SAUCES	Mayonnaise, imitation 1 tbsp	3
DAIRY	Milk, lofat, 1%, no addedsolid1 cup	3
SOUPS	Minestrone soup, canned 1 cup	3
SOUPS	Pea, green, soup, canned 1 cup	3

CHART BY FAT GRAMS

	Food	Fat Grams
NUTS	Popcorn, popped, veg oil,saltd1 cup	3
MEATS	Pork, luncheon meat,ckd ham,ln2 slices	3
VEGETABLES	Refried beans, canned 1 cup	3
BREADS	Rolls, dinner, home recipe 1 roll	3
BREADS	Sandwich spread, pork, beef 1 tbsp	3
DAIRY	Sour cream 1 tbsp	3
VEGETABLES	Sweetpotatoes, candied 1 piece	3
POULTRY	Turkey ham, cured turkey thigh2 slices	3
POULTRY	Turkey, roasted, light meat 2 pieces	3
MEATS	Beef, dried, chipped 2.5 oz	4
BREADS	Bran muffins, from commerl mix1 muffin	4
SWEETS	Brownies w/ nuts,frstng,cmmrcl1 browne	4
DAIRY	Butter, salted 1 pat	4
DAIRY	Butter, unsalted 1 pat	4
POULTRY	Chicken roll, light 2 slices	4
VEGETABLES	Chickpeas, cooked, drained 1 cup	4
BREADS	Cornmeal,bolted,dry form 1 cup	4
DAIRY	Cottage cheese,lowfat 2% 1 cup	4
SWEETS	Devil's food cake,chocfrst,fmx1 cupcak	4
SWEETS	Fig bars 4 cookie	4
SWEETS	Gingerbread cake, from mix 1 piece	4
SAUCES	Gravy and turkey, frozen 5 oz	4
BREADS	Italian bread 1 loaf	4
DAIRY	Margarine, regulr,hard,80% fat1 pat	4
FISH	Oysters, raw 1 cup	4
MEATS	Pork, cured, bacon,canadn,cked2 slice	4
MEATS	Pork, cured, ham, rosted,lean 2.4 oz	4
MEATS	Pork, link, cooked 1 link	4
VEGETABLES	Potatoes,french-frd,frzn,oven 10 strip	4
DAIRY	Pudding, choc, cooked from mix1/2 cup	4
DAIRY	Pudding, choc, instant, fr mix1/2 cup	4
DAIRY	Pudding, rice, from mix 1/2 cup	4
DAIRY	Pudding, tapioca, from mix 1/2 cup	4
DAIRY	Pudding, vnlla,cooked from mix1/2 cup	4
DAIRY	Pudding, vnlla,instant frm mix1/2 cup	4
SPICES	Sesame seeds 1 tbsp	4
SWEETS	Sherbet, 2% fat 1 cup	4
SWEETS	Snack cakes,devils food,cremflsm cake	4
POULTRY	Turkey, roasted, light + dark 3 pieces	4
MEATS	Vienna sausage 1 sausag	4
DAIRY	Yogurt, w/ lofat milk, plain 8 oz	4

CHART BY FAT GRAMS

Food		Fat Grams
BREADS	Baking pwdr biscuits,homerecpe1 biscut	5
SAUCES	Beef gravy, canned 1 cup	5
MEATS	Beef heart, braised 3 oz	5
MEATS	Beef roast, eye o rnd, lean 2.6 oz	5
SWEETS	Blueberry muffins, home recipe1 muffin	5
SWEETS	Blueberry muffins,from com mix1 muffin	5
BREADS	Breadcrumbs, dry, grated 1 cup	5
MEATS	Brown and serve sausage,brwnd 1 link	5
BEVERAGES	Chocolate milk, lowfat 2% 1 cup	5
BREADS	Cornmeal,whole-grnd,unbolt,dry1 cup	5
DAIRY	Eggs, cooked, hard-cooked 1 egg	5
DAIRY	Eggs, cooked, poached 1 egg	5
DAIRY	Eggs, raw, whole 1 egg	5
DAIRY	Eggs, raw, yolk 1 yolk	5
DAIRY	Ice cream, vanlla, regulr 11% 3 fl oz	5
DAIRY	Ice milk, vanilla,softserv 3% 1 cup	5
DAIRY	Margarine, imitation 40% fat 1 tbsp	5
SAUCES	Mayonnaise type salad dressing1 tbsp	5
DAIRY	Milk, lofat, 2%, added solids 1 cup	5
DAIRY	Milk, lofat, 2%, no addedsolid1 cup	5
DAIRY	Mozzarella chese,skim, lomoist1 oz	5
CEREAL	Nature valley granola cereal 1 oz	5
VEGETABLES	Onion rings, breaded,frzn,prpd2 rings	5
FISH	Oysters, breaded, fried 1 oyster	5
SWEETS	Pound cake, commercial 1 slice	5
SWEETS	Pound cake, from home recipe 1 slice	5
DAIRY	Pudding, tapioca, canned 5 oz	5
FISH	Salmon, baked, red 3 oz	5
FISH	Salmon, canned, pink, w/ bones3 oz	5
SWEETS	Snack cakes,sponge creme fllngsm cake	5
SWEETS	Syrup, chocolate flvred, fudge2 tbsp	5
DAIRY	Tofu 1 piece	5
POULTRY	Turkey roast, frzn,lght+drk,ck3 oz	5
DAIRY	Whipping cream, unwhiped,light1 tbsp	5
CEREAL	100% natural cereal 1 oz	6
SAUCES	1000 island, salad drsng,reglr1 tbsp	6
VEGETABLES	Bean with bacon soup, canned 1 cup	6
MEATS	Beef steak,sirloin,broil,lean 2.5 oz	6
BREADS	Bran muffins, home recipe 1 muffin	6
SWEETS	Brownies w/ nuts,frm home recp1 browne	6
DAIRY	Cheddar cheese 1 cu in	6

CHART BY FAT GRAMS

	Food	Fat Grams
BREADS	Corn muffins, from commerl mix1 muffin	6
BREADS	Danish pastry, plain, no nuts 1 oz	6
DAIRY	Feta cheese 1 oz	6
FISH	Flounder or sole, baked, buttr3 oz	6
FISH	Flounder or sole, baked,margrn3 oz	6
FISH	Halibut, broiled, butter,lemju3 oz	6
DAIRY	Ice milk, vanilla, 4% fat 1 cup	6
MEATS	Lamb,chops,loin,broil,lean 2.3 oz	6
MEATS	Lamb,leg,roasted, lean only 2.6 oz	6
DAIRY	Mozzarella cheese, whole milk 1 oz	6
SAUCES	Mushroom gravy, canned 1 cup	6
DAIRY	Pasterzd proces chese spred,am1 oz	6
MEATS	Pork, luncheon meat,ckd ham,rg2 slices	6
BREADS	Toaster pastries 1 pastry	6
SOUPS	Tomato soup with milk, canned 1 cup	6
POULTRY	Turkey, roasted, dark meat 4 pieces	6
DAIRY	Whipping cream, unwhiped,heavy1 tbsp	6
VEGETABLES	Beans,dry,canned,w/pork+tomsce1 cup	7
MEATS	Beef liver, fried 3 oz	7
DAIRY	Buttermilk, dried 1 cup	7
POULTRY	Chicken, fried, flour, drmstck1.7 oz	7
SOUPS	Clam chowder, new eng, w/ milk1 cup	7
BREADS	Coffeecake, crumb, from mix 1 piece	7
SOUPS	Cr of chicken soup w/ h20,cnnd1 cup	7
DAIRY	Eggs, cooked, fried 1 egg	7
DAIRY	Eggs, cooked, scrambled/omelet1 egg	7
BREADS	French toast, home recipe 1 slice	7
SWEETS	Fruitcake,dark, from homerecip1 piece	7
MEATS	Lamb, rib, roasted, lean only 2 oz	7
MEATS	Lamb,chops,arm,braised,lean 1.7 oz	7
SWEETS	Milk chocolate candy,w/ rice c1 oz	7
DAIRY	Pasterzd proces cheese, swiss 1 oz	7
DAIRY	Pasterzd proces chese food,amr1 oz	7
MEATS	Pork, cured, ham, canned,roast3 oz	7
MEATS	Pork, luncheon meat,choppd ham2 slices	7
BREADS	Potato chips 10 chips	7
MEATS	Salami, dry type 2 slices	7
FISH	Tuna, cannd, drnd,oil,chk,lght3 oz	7
POULTRY	Turkey, roasted, light + dark 1 cup	7
SWEETS	Vanilla wafers 10 cooke	7
DAIRY	Yogurt, w/ whole milk 8 oz	7

CHART BY FAT GRAMS

	Food		Fat Grams
MEATS	Beef, ckd,bttm round,lean only	2.8 oz	8
DAIRY	Blue cheese	1 oz	8
SAUCES	Blue cheese salad dressing	1 tbsp	8
BEVERAGES	Chocolate milk, regular	1 cup	8
DAIRY	Cottage cheese,cremd,w/fruit	1 cup	8
SWEETS	Devil's food cake,chocfrst,fmx	1 piece	8
DAIRY	Milk, whole, 3.3% fat	1 cup	8
NUTS	Peanut butter	1 tbsp	8
MEATS	Pork chop, loin, broil, lean	2.5 oz	8
MEATS	Pork fresh ham, roastd, lean	2.5 oz	8
MEATS	Pork shoulder, braisd, lean	2.4 oz	8
VEGETABLES	Potatoes,french-frd,frzn,fried	10 strip	8
DAIRY	Provolone cheese	1 oz	8
BREADS	Rolls, hoagie or submarine	1 roll	8
FISH	Salmon, smoked	3 oz	8
SWEETS	Sandwich type cookie	4 cookie	8
DAIRY	Shakes, thick, chocolate	10 oz	8
SWEETS	Shortbread cookie, commercial	4 cookie	8
SWEETS	Shortbread cookie, home recipe	2 cookie	8
DAIRY	Swiss cheese	1 oz	8
SAUCES	Tartar sauce	1 tbsp	8
SAUCES	Vinegar and oil salad dressing	1 tbsp	8
BREADS	Waffles, from mix	1 waffle	8
SWEETS	Yellow cake w/ choc frst,frmix	1 piece	8
MEATS	Beef roast, rib, lean only	2.2 oz	9
MEATS	Beef, ckd,chuck blade,leanonly	2.2 oz	9
DAIRY	Camembert cheese	1 wedge	9
DAIRY	Cheddar cheese	1 oz	9
POULTRY	Chicken frankfurter	1 frank	9
POULTRY	Chicken, fried, flour, breast	3.5 oz	9
POULTRY	Chicken, stewed, light + dark	1 cup	9
SWEETS	Chocolate chip cookies,commrcl	4 cookie	9
SWEETS	Coca pwdr w/o nofat drymlk,prd	1 servng	9
BREADS	Corn chips	1 oz	9
DAIRY	Cottage cheese,cremd,smll curd	1 cup	9
SOUPS	Cr of mushrom soup w/ h2o,cnnd	1 cup	9
SAUCES	French salad dressing, regular	1 tbsp	9
FISH	Haddock, breaded, fried	3 oz	9
SAUCES	Italian salad dressing,regular	1 tbsp	9
DAIRY	Malted milk,chocolate, pwdrppd	1 servng	9
DAIRY	Margarine, spread,hard,60% fat	1 tbsp	9

CHART BY FAT GRAMS

Food		Fat Grams
DAIRY	Margarine, spread,soft,60% fat1 tbsp	9
SWEETS	Milk chocolate candy, plain 1 oz	9
DAIRY	Muenster cheese 1 oz	9
DAIRY	Parmesan cheese, grated 1 oz	9
DAIRY	Pasterzd proces cheese,americn1 oz	9
BREADS	Pizza, cheese 1 slice	9
MEATS	Pork, cured, bacon, regul,cked3 slice	9
VEGETABLES	Potatoes, mashed,recpe,mlk+mar1 cup	9
VEGETABLES	Potatoes, scalloped, home recp1 cup	9
FISH	Sardines, atlntc,cnned,oil,drn3 oz	9
DAIRY	Shakes, thick, vanilla 10 oz	9
PASTA	Spaghetti, tom sauce chee,hmrp1 cup	9
FISH	Trout, broiled, w/ buttr,lemju3 oz	9
MEATS	Veal cutlet, med fat,brsd,brld3 oz	9
SWEETS	White cake w/ wht frstng,comml1 piece	9
MEATS	Beef, canned, corned 3 oz	10
POULTRY	Chicken chow mein, home recipe1 cup	10
DAIRY	Cottage cheese,cremd,lrge curd1 cup	10
DAIRY	Cream cheese 1 oz	10
DAIRY	Imitatn whipd toping,pwdrd,prp1 cup	10
PASTA	Macaroni and cheese, canned 1 cup	10
DAIRY	Malted milk,natural, pwdr pprd1 servng	10
SWEETS	Milk chocolate candy,w/ almond1 oz	10
BREADS	Oatmeal w/ raisins cookies 4 cookie	10
MEATS	Pork fresh rib, roastd, lean 2.5 oz	10
VEGETABLES	Potatoes, au gratin, from mix 1 cup	10
DAIRY	Pudding, vanilla, canned 5 oz	10
FISH	Scallops, breaded, frzn,reheat6 scalop	10
FISH	Shrimp, french fried 3 oz	10
SAUCES	Soybeans, dry, cooked, drained1 cup	10
PASTA	Spaghetti,meatballs,tomsac,cnd1 cup	10
SWEETS	Sweet (dark) chocolate 1 oz	10
MEATS	Beef and vegetable stew,hm rcp1 cup	11
DAIRY	Butter, salted 1 tbsp	11
DAIRY	Butter, unsalted 1 tbsp	11
POULTRY	Chicken, canned, boneless 5 oz	11
POULTRY	Chicken, fried, batter,drmstck2.5 oz	11
SWEETS	Chocolate chip cookies,hme rcp4 cookie	11
SWEETS	Chocolate chip cookies,refrig 4 cookie	11
SOUPS	Cr of chicken soup w/ mlk,cnnd1 cup	11
MEATS	Hamburger, regular 1 sandwh	11

CHART BY FAT GRAMS

Food		Fat Grams
DAIRY	Margarine, regulr,hard,80% fat1 tbsp	11
DAIRY	Margarine, regulr,soft,80% fat1 tbsp	11
SAUCES	Mayonnaise, regular 1 tbsp	11
SWEETS	Milk chocolate candy,w/ penuts1 oz	11
PASTA	Noodles, chow mein, canned 1 cup	11
FISH	Ocean perch, breaded, fried 1 fillet	11
MEATS	Pork chop, loin,panfry, lean 2.4 oz	11
VEGETABLES	Potatoes, scalloped, from mix 1 cup	11
DAIRY	Pudding, chocolate,canned 5 oz	11
MEATS	Salami, cooked type 2 slices	11
BREADS	Taco 1 taco	11
SWEETS	Yellowcake w/ chocfrstng,comml1 piece	11
VEGETABLES	Beans,dry,canned,w/pork+swtsce1 cup	12
MEATS	Beef roast, eye o rnd,lean+fat3 oz	12
BREADS	Croissants 1 crosst	12
BREADS	Danish pastry, plain, no nuts 1 pastry	12
SWEETS	Doughnuts, cake type, plain 1 donut	12
VEGETABLES	Potatoes, mashed,frm dehydrted1 cup	12
SWEETS	Sheetcake,w/o frstng,homerecip1 piece	12
PASTA	Spaghetti,meatballs,tomsa,hmrp1 cup	12
SWEETS	Sugar cookie, from refrig dogh4 cookie	12
POULTRY	Turkey patties, brd,battd,frid1 patty	12
MEATS	Beef, ckd,bttm round,lean+ fat3 oz	13
NUTS	Cashew nuts, dry roastd,salted1 oz	13
NUTS	Cashew nuts, dry roastd,unsalt1 oz	13
BREADS	Danish pastry, fruit 1 pastry	13
SWEETS	Doughnuts, yeast-leavend,glzed1 donut	13
SAUCES	Fats, cooking/vegetbl shorteng1 tbsp	13
MEATS	Frankfurter, cooked 1 frank	13
FISH	Herring, pickled 3 oz	13
MEATS	Lamb,leg,roasted, lean+ fat 3 oz	13
DAIRY	Lard 1 tbsp	13
MEATS	Pork, luncheon meat,canned 2 slices	13
VEGETABLES	Pumpkin and squash kernels 1 oz	13
MEATS	Roast beef sandwich 1 sandwh	13
BREADS	Waffles, from home recipe 1 waffle	13
DAIRY	Whipped topping, pressurized 1 cup	13
SWEETS	White sauce w/ milk from mix 1 cup	13
NUTS	Cashew nuts, oil roastd,salted1 oz	14
NUTS	Cashew nuts, oil roastd,unsalt1 oz	14
SAUCES	Chicken gravy, canned 1 cup	14

CHART BY FAT GRAMS

	Food		Fat Grams
SAUCES	Corn oil	1 tbsp	14
SOUPS	Cr of mushrom soup w/ mlk,cnnd	1 cup	14
SWEETS	Fried pie, apple	1 pie	14
SWEETS	Fried pie, cherry	1 pie	14
DAIRY	Ice cream, vanlla, regulr 11%	1 cup	14
SWEETS	Lemon meringue pie	1 piece	14
SAUCES	Olive oil	1 tbsp	14
NUTS	Peanut butter cookie,home recp	4 cookie	14
SAUCES	Peanut oil	1 tbsp	14
NUTS	Peanuts, oil roasted, salted	1 oz	14
NUTS	Peanuts, oil roasted, unsalted	1 oz	14
NUTS	Pistachio nuts	1 oz	14
MEATS	Pork, cured, ham, rosted,ln+ft	3 oz	14
OILS	Safflower oil	1 tbsp	14
SWEETS	Sheetcake,w/ whfrstng,homercip	1 piece	14
SAUCES	Soybean oil, hydrogenated	1 tbsp	14
SAUCES	Soybean-cottonseed oil, hydrgn	1 tbsp	14
OILS	Sunflower oil	1 tbsp	14
NUTS	Sunflower seeds	1 oz	14
MEATS	Veal rib, med fat, roasted	3 oz	14
NUTS	Almonds, whole	1 oz	15
MEATS	Beef steak,sirloin,broil,ln+ft	3 oz	15
MEATS	Cheeseburger, regular	1 sandwh	15
SWEETS	Chocolate, bitter ot baking	1 oz	15
SWEETS	Coconut, raw, piece	1 piece	15
SWEETS	Custard, baked	1 cup	15
MEATS	Lamb,chops,arm,braised,lean+ft	2.2 oz	15
NUTS	Mixed nuts w/ peants,dry,saltd	1 oz	15
NUTS	Mixed nuts w/ peants,dry,unslt	1 oz	15
MEATS	Bologna	2 slices	16
VEGETABLES	Chili con carne w/ beans, cnnd	1 cup	16
BREADS	Cracked-wheat bread	1 loaf	16
BREADS	Enchilada	1 enchld	16
MEATS	Ground beef, broiled, lean	3 oz	16
DAIRY	Imitatn whipd toping,pressrzd	1 cup	16
MEATS	Lamb,chops,loin,broil,lean+fat	2.8 oz	16
NUTS	Mixed nuts w/ peants,oil,saltd	1 oz	16
NUTS	Mixed nuts w/ peants,oil,unslt	1 oz	16
BREADS	Pumpernickel bread	1 loaf	16
NUTS	Walnuts, black, chopped	1 oz	16
SWEETS	Blueberry pie	1 piece	17

CHART BY FAT GRAMS

	Food		Fat Grams
DAIRY	Cheese sauce w/ milk, frm mix 1 cup		17
MEATS	Chop suey w/ beef + pork,hmrcp1 cup		17
SWEETS	Custard pie	1 piece	17
BREADS	Mixed grain bread	1 loaf	17
SWEETS	Peach pie	1 piece	17
NUTS	Pine nuts	1 oz	17
SWEETS	Pumpkin pie	1 piece	17
BREADS	Rye bread, light	1 loaf	17
SWEETS	Apple pie	1 piece	18
VEGETABLES	Beans,dry,canned,w/frankfurter1 cup		18
MEATS	Braunschweiger	2 slices	18
SWEETS	Cheesecake	1 piece	18
SWEETS	Cherry pie	1 piece	18
POULTRY	Chicken and noodles, home recp1 cup		18
POULTRY	Chicken, fried, batter, breast4.9 oz		18
BREADS	Eng muffin, egg, cheese, bacon1 sandwh		18
NUTS	Filberts, (hazelnuts) chopped 1 oz		18
BREADS	French or vienna bread	1 loaf	18
MEATS	Ground beef, broiled, regular 3 oz		18
MEATS	Pork fresh ham, roastd,lean+ft3 oz		18
VEGETABLES	Potatoes, hashed brown,fr frzn1 cup		18
BREADS	Raisin bread	1 loaf	18
VEGETABLES	Spinach souffle	1 cup	18
NUTS	Walnuts, english, pieces	1 oz	18
BREADS	White bread	1 loaf	18
NUTS	Brazil nuts	1 oz	19
BEVERAGES	Eggnog	1 cup	19
BEVERAGES	Evaporated milk, whole, canned1 cup		19
DAIRY	Imitation whipped topping,frzn1 cup		19
NUTS	Pecans, halves	1 oz	19
MEATS	Pork chop, loin, broil, len+ft3.1 oz		19
VEGETABLES	Potatoes, au gratin, home recp1 cup		19
DAIRY	Ricotta cheese, part skim milk1 cup		19
FISH	Tuna salad	1 cup	19
BREADS	Wheat bread	1 loaf	19
SAUCES	Hollandaise sce, w/ h2o,frm mx1 cup		20
BREADS	Oatmeal bread	1 loaf	20
MEATS	Pork fresh rib, roastd,lean+ft3 oz		20
SWEETS	Whole-wheat bread	1 loaf	20
SWEETS	Carrot cake,cremchese frst,rec1 piece		21
MEATS	Hamburger, 4oz patty	1 sandwh	21

CHART BY FAT GRAMS

	Food	Fat Grams
VEGETABLES	Potato salad made w/ mayonnais1 cup	21
NUTS	Macadamia nuts, oilrstd,salted1 oz	22
NUTS	Macadamia nuts, oilrstd,unsalt1 oz	22
PASTA	Macaroni and cheese, home rcpe1 cup	22
MEATS	Pork shoulder, braisd,lean+fat3 oz	22
SWEETS	Creme pie 1 piece	23
FISH	Fish sandwich, reg, w/ cheese 1 sandwh	23
DAIRY	Ice cream, vanlla, soft serve 1 cup	23
DAIRY	Ice cream, vanlla, rich 16% ft1 cup	24
POULTRY	Duck, roasted, flesh only 1/2 duck	25
MEATS	Beef roast, rib, lean + fat 3 oz	26
MEATS	Beef, ckd,chuck blade,lean+fat3 oz	26
BREADS	Bread stuffing,from mx,moist 1 cup	26
MEATS	Lamb, rib, roasted, lean + fat3 oz	26
VEGETABLES	Avocados, florida 1 avocdo	27
SWEETS	Coconut, raw, shredded 1 cup	27
FISH	Fish sandwich, lge, w/o cheese1 sandwh	27
MEATS	Pork chop, loin,panfry,lean+ft3.1 oz	27
SWEETS	Sweetened condensed milk cnnd 1 cup	27
BEVERAGES	Half and half, cream 1 cup	28
VEGETABLES	Avocados, california 1 avocdo	30
MEATS	Beef potpie, home recipe 1 piece	30
DAIRY	Parmesan cheese, grated 1 cup	30
SWEETS	White sauce, medium, home recp1 cup	30
BREADS	Bread stuffing,from mx,drytype1 cup	31
MEATS	Cheeseburger, 4oz patty 1 sandwh	31
POULTRY	Chicken potpie, home recipe 1 piece	31
SWEETS	Sherbet, 2% fat 1/2 gal	31
SWEETS	Pecan pie 1 piece	32
DAIRY	Ricotta cheese, whole milk 1 cup	32
SWEETS	Coconut, dried, sweetnd,shredd1 cup	33
POULTRY	Chicken a la king, home recipe1 cup	34
DAIRY	Chedddar cheese, shredded 1 cup	37
SWEETS	Gingerbread cake, from mix 1 cake	39
DAIRY	Imitatn sour dressing 1 cup	39
BREADS	Coffeecake, crumb, from mix 1 cake	41
DAIRY	Ice milk, vanilla, 4% fat 1/2 gal	45
DAIRY	Light, coffee or table cream 1 cup	46
DAIRY	Quiche lorraine 1 slice	48
DAIRY	Sour cream 1 cup	48
BREADS	Piecrust,from home recipe 1 shell	60

CHART BY FAT GRAMS

Food			Fat Grams
SWEETS	Semisweet chocolate	1 cup	61
NUTS	Cashew nuts, dry roastd,unsalt	1 cup	63
NUTS	Cashew nuts, dry roasted,saltd	1 cup	63
NUTS	Cashew nuts, oil roastd,salted	1 cup	63
NUTS	Cashew nuts, oil roastd,unsalt	1 cup	63
DAIRY	Margarine, spread,hard,60% fat	1/2 cup	69
NUTS	Almonds, slivered	1 cup	70
BREADS	Danish pastry, plain, no nuts	1 ring	71
NUTS	Peanuts, oil roasted, salted	1 cup	71
NUTS	Peanuts, oil roasted, unsalted	1 cup	71
NUTS	Walnuts, black, chopped	1 cup	71
NUTS	Filberts, (hazelnuts) chopped	1 cup	72
NUTS	Pecans, halves	1 cup	73
NUTS	Walnuts, english, pieces	1 cup	74
DAIRY	Whipping cream, unwhiped,light	1 cup	74
SWEETS	Lemon meringue pie	1 pie	86
DAIRY	Margarine, imitation 40% fat	8 oz	88
DAIRY	Whipping cream, unwhiped,heavy	1 cup	88
DAIRY	Margarine, regulr,hard,80% fat	1/2 cup	91
DAIRY	Butter, salted	1/2 cup	92
DAIRY	Butter, unsalted	1/2 cup	92
BREADS	Piecrust, from mix	2 crust	93
SWEETS	Pound cake, commercial	1 loaf	94
SWEETS	Pound cake, from home recipe	1 loaf	94
SWEETS	Custard pie	1 pie	101
SWEETS	Peach pie	1 pie	101
SWEETS	Blueberry pie	1 pie	102
SWEETS	Pumpkin pie	1 pie	102
NUTS	Macadamia nuts, oilrstd,salted	1 cup	103
NUTS	Macadamia nuts, oilrstd,unsalt	1 cup	103
SWEETS	Apple pie	1 pie	105
SWEETS	Cherry pie	1 pie	107
SWEETS	Sheetcake w/o frstng,homerecip	1 cake	108
DAIRY	Ice cream, vanlla, regulr 11%	1/2 galn	115
SWEETS	Yellow cake w/ choc frst,frmix	1 cake	125
SWEETS	Sheetcake,w/ whfrstng,homercip	1 cake	129
SWEETS	Devil's food cake,chocfrst,fmx	1 cake	136
DAIRY	Margarine, spread,soft,60% fat	8 oz	138
SWEETS	Creme pie	1 pie	139
SWEETS	White cake w/ wht frstng,comml	1 cake	148
SWEETS	Yellowcake w/ chocfrstng,comml	1 cake	175

CHART BY FAT GRAMS

	Food	Fat Grams
DAIRY	Margarine, regulr,soft,80% fat8 oz	183
SWEETS	Pecan pie 1 pie	189
DAIRY	Ice cream, vanlla, rich 16% ft1/2 gal	190
SAUCES	Fats, cooking/vegetbl shorteng1 cup	205
DAIRY	Lard 1 cup	205
SWEETS	Cheesecake 1 cake	213
SAUCES	Olive oil 1 cup	216
SAUCES	Peanut oil 1 cup	216
SAUCES	Corn oil 1 cup	218
OILS	Safflower oil 1 cup	218
SAUCES	Soybean oil, hydrogenated 1 cup	218
SAUCES	Soybean-cottonseed oil, hydrgn1 cup	218
OILS	Sunflower oil 1 cup	218
SWEETS	Fruitcake,dark, from homerecip1 cake	228
SWEETS	Carrot cake,cremchese frst,rec1 cake	328

MY OWN FOODS AND NOTES

MY OWN FOODS AND NOTES

FOOD   FAT   CARBS   CALORIES

_____   _____   _____   _____

_____   _____   _____   _____

_____   _____   _____   _____

_____   _____   _____   _____

_____   _____   _____   _____

_____   _____   _____   _____

_____   _____   _____   _____

_____   _____   _____   _____

_____   _____   _____   _____

_____   _____   _____   _____

_____   _____   _____   _____

_____   _____   _____   _____

_____   _____   _____   _____

_____   _____   _____   _____

_____   _____   _____   _____

_____   _____   _____   _____

_____   _____   _____   _____

_____   _____   _____   _____

MY OWN FOODS AND NOTES

FOOD   FAT   CARBS   CALORIES

_____   _____   _____   _____

_____   _____   _____   _____

_____   _____   _____   _____

_____   _____   _____   _____

_____   _____   _____   _____

_____   _____   _____   _____

_____   _____   _____   _____

_____   _____   _____   _____

_____   _____   _____   _____

_____   _____   _____   _____

_____   _____   _____   _____

_____   _____   _____   _____

_____   _____   _____   _____

_____   _____   _____   _____

_____   _____   _____   _____

_____   _____   _____   _____

_____   _____   _____   _____

_____   _____   _____   _____

MY OWN FOODS AND NOTES

FOOD   FAT   CARBS   CALORIES

_____   _____ _____ _____

_____   _____ _____ _____

_____   _____ _____ _____

_____   _____ _____ _____

_____   _____ _____ _____

_____   _____ _____ _____

_____   _____ _____ _____

_____   _____ _____ _____

_____   _____ _____ _____

_____   _____ _____ _____

_____   _____ _____ _____

_____   _____ _____ _____

_____   _____ _____ _____

_____   _____ _____ _____

_____   _____ _____ _____

_____   _____ _____ _____

_____   _____ _____ _____

_____   _____ _____ _____

_____   _____ _____ _____

MY OWN FOODS AND NOTES

FOOD   FAT   CARBS   CALORIES

FOOD	FAT	CARBS	CALORIES

MY OWN FOODS AND NOTES

FOOD

FAT CARBS CALORIES

_____   _____ _____ _____

_____   _____ _____ _____

_____   _____ _____ _____

_____   _____ _____ _____

_____   _____ _____ _____

_____   _____ _____ _____

_____   _____ _____ _____

_____   _____ _____ _____

_____   _____ _____ _____

_____   _____ _____ _____

_____   _____ _____ _____

_____   _____ _____ _____

_____   _____ _____ _____

_____   _____ _____ _____

_____   _____ _____ _____

_____   _____ _____ _____

_____   _____ _____ _____

NOTES

NOTES

NOTES

NOTES

www.ingramcontent.com/pod-product-compliance
Lightning Source LLC
Chambersburg PA
CBHW080047280326
41934CB00014B/3241